Praise for E.N.D. the Diet Drama
previously titled *Join Me in the END Zone*

"Ashly is a master at utilizing her experience, wisdom and passion to ensure her clients achieve life changing results. In this book she provides, quite literally, a recipe for success and a multi-faceted approach in support of the body, mind *and* soul to live a life of balance and harmony in a body that you love. Sharing her real-life experiences, Ashly walks with you along the journey of uncovering and discovering the necessary elements for you to achieve a life-long transformation from inside and out.

In creating anything in life, it *always* begins with the first step. What I know for sure, is that you are holding the keys to finally ***E.N.D the Diet Drama, Lose the Weight and Reclaim Your Life*** - and your journey begins here!"

Patricia Barnett
International Best-Selling Author
Wealth Mastery for Women - 12 Laws to Create Wealth Starting Today

"Ashly Torian's *Join Me in the END Zone* is a marriage of brilliant, soul-opening perspectives and actionable, real steps a person can take to find a refreshing new approach to a very old problem—weight and body issues. Ashly uses her own struggles to inspire, teach and motivate us to step back and simply consider a different idea. This book is a bright light in the world of health and weight loss advice!"

Cynthia Stadd
Eating Psychology Practitioner and Speaker

"This is a 5-Star book! I love the way Ashly gives readers practical ways to not only manage their weight, but to feed their souls as well. I recommend this book with two enthusiastic thumbs up!"

Dr. Paula Fellingham,
Global Mentor for Women www.TotalLifeExcellence.com

Balboa Press books may be ordered through booksellers or by contacting:

Balboa Press
A Division of Hay House
1663 Liberty Drive
Bloomington, IN 47403
www.balboapress.com
1 (877) 407-4847

Because of the dynamic nature of the Internet, any web addresses or links contained in this book may have changed since publication and may no longer be valid. The views expressed in this work are solely those of the author and do not necessarily reflect the views of the publisher, and the publisher hereby disclaims any responsibility for them.

The author of this book does not dispense medical advice or prescribe the use of any technique as a form of treatment for physical, emotional, or medical problems without the advice of a physician, either directly or indirectly. The intent of the author is only to offer information of a general nature to help you in your quest for emotional and spiritual well-being. In the event you use any of the information in this book for yourself, which is your constitutional right, the author and the publisher assume no responsibility for your actions.

Any people depicted in stock imagery provided by Thinkstock are models, and such images are being used for illustrative purposes only.
Certain stock imagery © Thinkstock.

Print information available on the last page.

ISBN: 978-1-5043-9021-7 (sc)
ISBN: 978-1-5043-9023-1 (hc)
ISBN: 978-1-5043-9022-4 (e)

Library of Congress Control Number: 2017916930

Balboa Press rev. date: 11/10/2017

Cover and book design by Brooke Hawkins Design
www.brookehawkins.myportfolio.com

Photography by Cathy Lynn Vernon

To protect the privacy of my clients, the personal stories related in this book, while based on my experiences, are offered as illustrations and should not be construed as representing any particular person.

This book is intended as an informational guide to healthy living. The techniques described are meant to supplement, and are not a substitute for professional medical care or treatment. They should not be used to treat a serious ailment without prior consultation with a qualified healthcare professional.

Real Food Technology, Ambrotose and Mannatech are trademarks of Mannatech Incorporated and are used with permission.

Note from the Author

During its first run, *Join Me in the E.N.D. Zone* was a big hit! Due to the masculine nature of the title, women were not as drawn to the book as men. Because of this, I changed the title to:

E.N.D. the Diet Drama
3 Keys to Lose the Weight & Reclaim Your Life
Embrace ~ Nourish ~ Digest

In my work, I guide men and women to lose the weight and reclaim their lives. What I know for sure, is my method certainly works for everyone and it will for you, too.

This new title speaks to both feminine and masculine natures. My desire is to encourage women and men to live inspired, healthy and free, in bodies they love, by E.N.D.ing the diet drama and reclaiming their lives.

My greatest wish is that by reading this book, you gain insight and knowledge regarding your own struggle with food, your health and body image, to ultimately find freedom on the other side.

Ashly Torian

Dedication

Mama, you have been there from the beginning, steadfast and true, always believing in me and investing in me with your time, love and wisdom. All I can say is, you are amazing, and I am the lucky one.

greatest teachers through my journey, not only in my personal transformation, but also in the development of programs that can transform others. Thank you for your trust in my abilities and your commitment to living a healthy and purpose-filled life.

To the One who rescued me, I will call on You the rest of my days.

"Embrace the moment you are in. Be present in your body and in your life." – Ashly

Behold the apple and marvel at its compact beauty—shiny, red, and smooth. Take a crisp bite. Taste the sweetness of the juice on the tongue, feel the firm texture in the mouth, and relish the orchard-fresh scent of this luscious fruit. Wonder at how this apple came to be in your hands: the sprouting of a single seed so many years ago, the appearance of a sapling on a warm spring day, the growth of a tree over many seasons of sun and rain, snow and heat. Take another bite. Mindfully consider those who patiently tended the orchard, pruned the trees, and picked this one particular apple from branches sagging with their bounty. Savor the natural sugars and be aware of the goodness about to nourish your body: vitamin C and nearly two dozen other vitamins, minerals, and organic compounds essential for cellular vitality. Consider the dietary fiber and its essential value in the digestive process. Chew, taste, and swallow. Behold the apple, and enjoy the singular miracle that is your life.

Foreword

In my journey to ultimate health, I found that not only what you eat and how you exercise makes a person healthy, but also what you feed your mind, your positive self-talk, and constantly reading and learning for your own self-improvement. Ashly Torian has helped hundreds of people lose weight, but has also helped to change their thinking about how they view themselves. She has the knowledge, tools and ability to help anyone get the results they want, both physically and mentally. By reading and studying this powerful book and following what Ashly teaches, you can change. You can improve. You will be motivated. You see, each of us has the ability to change our thoughts, change our actions, change our lives, and meet Ashly in the END Zone.

Tony Jeary
The RESULTS Guy™

- **E**mbrace the wonder that is your body.

- **N**ourish your body to fulfill your purpose.

- **D**igest the world around you, not only food and drink, but also the observations and lessons that make you who you are.

When you do these things thoughtfully and with awareness, you are in the **END Zone**, the time and place to maximize your wellbeing. The **END Zone** is not a weight-loss program. It's not a fad diet. But by entering the **END Zone**, you will lose the weight and it will stay off. If you are in an unhealthy relationship with food—perhaps you eat too much, or, conversely, too little— the **END Zone** will help you find the balance that's best for optimizing your body's potential. If you tend to be sedentary, or you drive yourself in high-intensity, until-you-drop workouts, the **END Zone** can provide the particular kind of fitness equilibrium that satisfies your needs.

That's because the **END Zone** is a mindset, a way to think about who you are, what you want to do, and the body you need to do it.

Do you want more out of life? Do you want to feel better, think more clearly, and have the energy to fulfill your dreams? If you want these things, then join me in the **END Zone**.

Contents

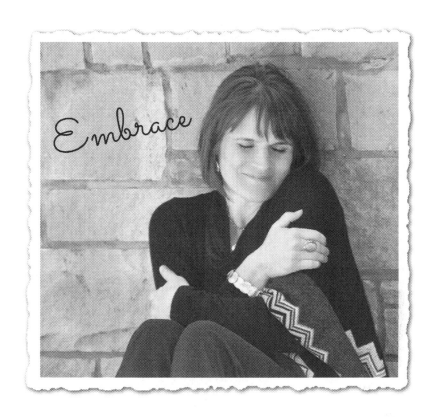

PART 1

"Love your body to get the body you love."—Ashly

1:

Learning to Appreciate My Temple

Ever since I can remember, I loved movement. When I was three, maybe four years old, I was amazed that my little body could do what I willed it to do, tumble, roll, leap, and run. I challenged my older sister and brother to driveway dashes and around-the-block marathons. It was intoxicating, feeling that adrenaline rush, discovering how my body could perform, and how I could draw from reserves deep inside to press on. Observing our backyard handstands, cartwheels, and somersaults, my parents purchased a gymnastics mat for our suburban Dallas home. When I turned five, they enrolled me in a noncompetitive beginner's gymnastics class at our local recreation center. It was fun learning the basics of floor exercise, uneven bars, the balance beam, and vault.

I was ten years old when a Romanian girl, who was only four years older than I, lit up the Montreal Summer Olympics. I wanted to be like Nadia Comaneci, earn perfect scores of 10, and wear gold medals around my neck. I was psyched to become a gymnastics champion. A competitive coach, well known in gymnastics circles around Texas, soon accepted me into his program. Among the ten girls in the class, I carried the most weight at 98 pounds.

At the start of each class, before we were allowed to hit the mats, the coach weighed us. It became a weekly ordeal I dreaded.

cuddled. Here I was, a sixth grade girl being rocked to sleep like an infant.

As I look back over this time in my life, I recognize that Dr. Solomon's "letter therapy" may seem a bit odd, but it worked. Avoiding the necessity of attending a special school, I was able to remain in my sixth grade classroom. My grades dramatically improved, and I was earning mostly Bs and some As. I could recall textbook material, follow directions, and communicate better. It wasn't that I lacked intelligence, rather I had a learning challenge, and it was corrected. When you have a struggle as a child, such as a learning disability, you discover a reserve of resilience deep down within yourself that prepares you for other life challenges.

This resilience was again tested on a two-week wilderness trek in the Rocky Mountains. Our church sponsored an annual summer youth trip, and since I was about to enter the ninth grade, I was now old enough to go. My sister Jamie, who is a year older than I, had taken this trip the previous year, and was a returning camper. This particular summer, our initial destination was Colorado's Great Sand Dunes National Park. In the San Luis Valley, at the base of the Sangre de Cristo Mountain Range, lies one of America's most amazing natural wonders, a windswept "high desert" terrain of sand with dunes towering more than 700 feet in height.

During our first week in Colorado, we were in "base camp," learning the basics such as hiking long distances, map reading, climbing, and top-rope belaying, the technique of scaling a mountain with ropes and harnesses. Bible studies rounded out the days. In the second week, we hiked the dunes, climbed to the summit of Medano Peak, elevation 13,135 feet, and stood on the grassy, tundra-like apex to view the magnificent snowcapped Rockies stretching to the horizon.

Volunteers joined a select group to scale a more challenging rock formation, one requiring a series of three-pitch climbs, each pitch 40 feet or more in height, straight up the vertical face of the mountain. Considered by the leaders as one of the stronger campers, I was on the first pitch, meaning I was on the bottom, about to belay two more campers up the rock face above me. I made a bite in the rope and looped the line through the locking carabiner, securing the rope to the harness around my waist. Gripping the climber's end of the rope above me with my left hand, or the guide hand, and the brake end of the rope with my right, I began pulling with my guide hand.

As the day drew long, belaying became more of an ordeal than a fun afternoon activity. I literally held a fellow climber's life in my hands, so there was no choice but to keep pulling, regardless of how my arms ached and muscles burned. My mantra became "persevere, keep going, and never give up." That night, my biceps were each swollen to the size of a grapefruit, but I felt strong, even invincible. I was gaining an appreciation for the temple that was my body.

*"Determine what is true within;
that truth does not vary. Life is what
varies, shifts, and changes form,
but truth does not change. Rely on it."*
—Ashly

2:

Temples, Warts & All

In the **END Zone**, we embrace ourselves, warts and all. The Christian Bible says our bodies are temples of the spirit that resides within us. (1 Corinthians 6:19-20) The Hindu belief is that the body serves as a temple for the soul, and the Supreme Being resides within the soul. Since I come from a Christian perspective, to me, the body is the vessel that carries the eternal spirit of God along with our soul, namely our will, conscience, and our ability to reason and think. Each of us is a three-part being comprised of the body, the soul, and the spirit, and of these three, the body is the part that brings tactile pleasure. To enjoy life to the fullest, we need to pay attention to our bodies, honor and respect them, because we have no replacements.

However, honor and respect do not mean we must strive to maintain the Hollywood film-star version of the perfect body. It does not mean restricting our foods to those considered "super nutritious." Extremes are seldom healthful. Fixating on the perfect Adonis or Aphrodite body can be as detrimental as gobbling bags of potato chips day and night.

Jennifer wanted the perfect body and believed the perfect diet was the way to get it. Every morsel that passed her lips had

all around you. Through your nose, take a deep breath. Relax the shoulders and, through your mouth, exhale. Inhale through the nose and exhale through the mouth. Expel all the stale air from the lungs. Again, take a deep breath in through your nose. Release it through your mouth. Remove all the stale air, and, when you do this, work the diaphragm and squeeze out the last bit of air from the lungs. Take in another breath through the nose and exhale through the nose.

Continue breathing deeply. Stimulate the nervous system. Bring your senses to life. Awaken the senses, home in on yourself, and feel what is happening within. Breathe in through the nose, feel the air come up through the nasal passage, down the back of the throat to the lungs, the diaphragm, and if you have difficulty bringing that breath all the way to the diaphragm, then place your hand over your heart and begin with heart breaths. Breathe in and bring the breath to the heart and exhale. The more you practice this, the deeper you will be able to go down into the diaphragm. As you take in a breath, allow yourself to start at your feet, and imagine that breath coming through the soles of your feet, up through your thighs, abdomen, the chest, all the way to the top of your head. Bring the oxygen to the brain, so it can circulate. Exhale.

Take that breath down through the back of your head, the neck, and across the shoulders. Relax the shoulders and let the oxygen flow out through your fingers. Again, visualize the breath coming in through the soles of your feet. Allow the next inhalation to rise through the legs, through the abdomen, and circulate through the abdomen, oxygenating the intestines, the digestive system, all the way up to the heart. Oxygenate the heart and up to the top of the head, and, as you exhale, feel your tension and pressure flow out with the oxygen down through your head, neck, chest, abdomen, the front of your thighs, and out the soles of your feet.

In the next inhalation, bring the breath through the soles of the feet, up through the back of the thighs, and let that oxygen circulate through the lower back. Let it gather at the tension points as it rises up through the spine to the top of the head. As you exhale, envision the tension released from your head all the way down to the neck, the back, the hips, the thighs, and out through the feet.

Continue with the visualization of the oxygen flowing up through the body and circulating back out through the body. As it does, the tension and stress will flow out through the soles of the feet. Sit there for a moment as you breathe in. Take a relaxed breath, and release the breath. Be mindful of any tension in the body. Feel the chest with your slow, deep breathing. Relax the shoulders. Relax the tension along the spine, the abdomen, the hips, and the feet. Let your body rest for a moment in total relaxation, peace, harmony, love, openness, awareness, and when you are ready, and you feel you are at your most relaxed state, open your eyes and take in your surroundings. Don't just see the leaves of the tree, but see the space between the leaves. Don't just see the birds flying through the air, but really look at the birds, the tilt of their wings. Even be aware of the pesky gnat, the way it flies in a spiral, flitting here and there. Allow life to slow down in front of you and take it all in. See what new sights are around you today. Allow the breath to flow into the body, and release the breath. Slow down the pace, and witness the unfolding of life before you. Take a deep breath in. Exhale.

Slowing down to mindfully breathe is helpful for anyone. For centuries, Eastern cultures have practiced these techniques, and today, we commonly refer to it as Yoga, a Sanskrit word meaning union, connection, and conjunction. Purposeful meditation and contemplation are known to reduce heart rate, lower blood pressure, and ease stress.

The breathing exercise, by its nature, is personal, so make it your own. Select locations that serve you well. If you are the type of person who schedules the day ahead, then of course, continue to schedule time for yourself. If you are a more spontaneous individual, enjoy this exercise when the moment is right. Whether it is scheduled or not, treat yourself to this practice often, if only a few minutes a day. Breathe with intention. Take pleasure in the awareness of your senses.

"Embrace your best self by reflecting well on what you see in the mirror."
—Ashly

3:

Mirror, Mirror, Show Me All

The Yoga-style breathing exercise brings you in communion with your senses. The mirror brings you in relationship with your body and soul. We use a mirror to go much deeper as we strive to embrace our bodies, our being, and purpose. If you do not already have a full-length mirror, please purchase one. An inexpensive back-of-the-door mirror is usually less than twenty dollars. With the mirror in place, and with clothes on, look at yourself for five to ten minutes. For many people, a good look in the mirror can be unsettling. They immediately focus on flaws, real or imagined, such as a nose they think is too large, a chin that protrudes too much, a neck that's not long enough, and on it goes. Isn't it interesting that we see the negatives before the positives? If you are nit-picking, only seeing imperfections, begin by looking at yourself in the eyes. Now, open a positive dialogue with the individual staring back at you. After all, if we intend to embrace our best selves, we should begin by speaking well of the reflections we see.

Say, "I love you." Tell yourself how important you are to you. Since the words we voice are reflections of our thoughts, reflect back into the mirror words of affirmation such as:

"I am alive, and I approve of whom I am."

"I accept myself just the way I am."

"I believe in me."

"I cherish who I am."

"I care about me and want the best for me."

"I am good, generous, and full of grace."

"I can accomplish anything I set my mind to do."

If you visited my home, you would find a series of about eight index cards taped around my mirror. On these cards, I have written affirmations that are like mantras to me. Here are some of them:

"I have time and space for all I need to do."

"I love and approve of myself. I'm at peace with myself. All is well."

"I release the past, so the new and vital will enter."

"I love the Lord, for He heard my voice and my cry for mercy."

Consider words of encouragement that are true for you at this moment in your life. What words of affirmation resonate with you? Use these thought-starters by filling in the statements:

"I know that I am…"

"Right now, at this moment in my life, I…"

"I choose to…"

"Yes, I am…"

I have found that affirmations that speak to me are those I feel deep inside myself. I repeat them often, let the words sink in, and the more I repeat them, the more energized I become. Feel your positive words. Let them speak to your heart, and let them reveal your heart to others.

Take time every day to "work the mirror." Like any newly learned skill, it requires time and practice, so don't give up if it all seems a bit awkward. Over a period of weeks, you will come to fully appreciate "you" for who you are, with or without clothes! You will fully value the temple that is your body, and feel blessed to have it, and when we love where we are at the moment, we can begin to love where we are going. Love the body you are in to get the body you love. When we have a love for ourselves, and are fully at ease within our bodies, we feel good about ourselves. We are prepared to embrace the present, so we can move on to the future.

Author Louise Hay in her 1984 book, *You Can Heal Your Life*, suggests "mirror talk," the use of positive affirmations, can help address emotional issues and physical maladies. In my experience, we can use our reflection in the mirror to come to terms with ourselves, appreciate our spiritual gifts, and discover our purpose in life. Each of us struggles with the fundamental questions of our existence: Why am I here? What is my purpose in life? What resonates in my heart?

The answers to these questions determine every part of you. Once you grasp your life's purpose, you will have the desire to make sure your body is in the shape it needs to be so you can fulfill your destiny.

Remember Jennifer, the health food junkie? Standing naked in front of a mirror, seeing her emaciated form brought her to tears. From childhood, she wished to dance. It was a desire that became a passion the day her mother took her to a New York performance of the American Ballet Theatre's *Romeo & Juliet*, featuring the internationally acclaimed Diana Vishneva. From that day on, Jennifer was driven to excel in ballet classes, training in Dallas and later in Vienna. Demanding the best for her body, this dancer's spiral into orthorexia started innocently enough. At first, she purged her diet of animal and dairy products, and then she tossed out anything made with artificial colors, flavors, or preservatives. The restrictions continued unabated until she was eating little more than raw homegrown vegetables, a few varieties of nuts, and a limited selection of whole grains. In her weak state, she could no longer continue dancing. By having her body write a letter to herself, applying the tenets of "mirror talk," and with coaching, Jennifer embraced her body. When she learned to listen to her body, it spoke to her. It wanted to live and again feel the thrill of the dance.

For Jennifer, coming to terms with her body meant reconnecting with her dream. She started to turn her life around when she decided to take in the nourishment her body required to fulfill her life's purpose and reason for being. With therapy, coaching, and professional counseling, she resumed her ballet career.

In much the same way, binge eaters Randy, Rachel, and Gabi each had a second chance to live their best lives. Randy has yet to hike the Appalachian Trail, but he connected with a "volkswalking" club, joining other enthusiasts for ten-kilometer hikes through historic sites, state preserves, and national parks. Rachel was able to regularly take her grandchildren to a community pool and playground. Gabi became a middle-school teacher and girls' volleyball coach.

However, for some individuals, the reasons they want to be fitter are not readily apparent.

"My sister is getting married next spring, and I'm the maid-of-honor," Rachel said.

"That's wonderful," I replied.

"No, it's not wonderful at all," she stated. "I need to lose eighty pounds. Can you get this weight off me in time? I have eight months before the wedding."

I made a quick calculation. "Eight months. That's forty weeks, or two pounds a week," I noted with a smile. "That's a very doable and safe weight-loss program."

That very day, we went to work, adjusting Rachel's diet, prescribing moderate daily aerobics and adding strength training twice a week. Gradually at first, and more steadily as the days progressed, she lost an average of two to three pounds a week. The following June, Rachel shared photos of her sister's wedding, and the bride was beautiful, but Rachel was radiant in her new, slimmer body.

powering our bodily functions, and, if there is excess food, storing it in the fat cells for later use. Yet, most of us will never need those excess food stores. As a result, an estimated seventy percent of the American adult population is overweight, and thirty-six percent is obese, meaning these individuals are carrying twenty percent or more pounds in weight that's not needed, weight stored as fat.

However, when we eat nutritious meals to fulfill our daily purpose, there's no need to store foods for times of scarcity. We eat what we need. No more. No less.

"But what about the really tasty things I can't live without?" you may ask. "Do you seriously want me to give up chocolate cake?"

Not at all. For example, I love ice cream, particularly homemade vanilla ice cream, made with plenty of eggs, heavy cream, and sugar. It's delicious, and, yes, I can't imagine not having it every so often, and that's the way I enjoy vanilla ice cream—every so often. I'll have my vanilla ice cream, not every day, but every so often, and not the entire tub, but a single scoop, enough to satisfy me. By the way, I will not settle for just any vanilla ice cream. If I'm having my scoop of vanilla, it's got to be the very best. When you have a craving for a less-than-healthy food, such as chocolate cake or vanilla ice cream, have a little, enough to satisfy the desire, and make it the best you can afford.

Eating to fulfill our life's purpose is more about quality than it is about quantity. For many years, I subscribed to the "calories in and calories out" school of weight gain versus weight loss. I was obsessed with counting every calorie I consumed, weighed myself on the scale several times daily, and was miserable. If I craved homemade vanilla ice cream or another "treat," I felt a wave of guilt. If I convinced myself that "everything in moderation" made sense and ate the "treat," the guilt was more palpable, so I deprived myself of some other food to counteract the calories. How many calories of fruits and veggies equal a bowl of ice cream? After all, calories are calories, right?

Wrong. The notion that all foods are created equal is nonsense. A calorie of ice cream is not the same as a calorie of broccoli. A way to measure the energy found in a lump of coal is no way to determine what we should or should not eat. Calorie counting is not only inadequate, but also counterproductive. The foods we consume, how the body reacts to them, and how they power us through the day are far more complex than burning coal to heat a steam engine.

Before consuming the 110 calories found in the dark chocolate granola snack bar, which is sold as a weight-management food, we should ask the question: Is this processed, packaged food benefiting the body as much as an apple or some other natural food? When it comes to losing pounds and maintaining a healthy weight, the Harvard School of Public Health wanted to know which was better: counting total calories, especially total fat and sugars, or counting on eating a healthy diet. Hands down, the study showed simply counting calories does not work and may be detrimental. The paper's lead author, Dr. Darius Mozaffarian, a cardiologist and epidemiologist at Harvard Medical School, noted consumers who select foods based on total calories may not be eating a diet that's best for overall health. For instance, instead of snacking on a serving of nuts containing 165 calories, we may instead down a can of soda containing 120 calories, thinking the fewer calories were better for us. Not so in this case. Nuts are known to help people reduce weight, while soda, rich in high-fructose corn syrup, is a contributor to weight gain. It's not about calories. It's about the food's impact on our bodily processes.

True or false: Since a serving of reduced-fat crackers has fewer calories (70) than a four-ounce serving of sweet potatoes (80), I can enjoy the better-tasting crackers and be healthier because I took in fewer calories.

FALSE. The crackers deny your body of healthy vegetable oils while sending starch and salt into your system. The sweet potato

5:

A Type-A's Ideal Relationships

At work, at home, or wherever she went, Theresa was a blur of motion. If ever there was a Type-A woman, it was this top corporate executive and single mother of two. At our first session, this new client told me about her career as the head of an auto parts manufacturing company's legal department. Divorced for the past six years and with two boys, one in middle school and the other a high school freshman, she spoke a mile-a-minute and seemed to be living life at a hundred-miles-an-hour clip. To keep ahead of her demanding job, she often ate meals at her desk. Here was the daily routine: Arriving at the office, Theresa had a breakfast of blueberry bagels with cream cheese or chocolate chip muffins and latte, placed on her desk by an executive assistant. At lunchtime, an intern was sent to fetch a fast food meal, usually a salad and soup, a chicken sandwich, or an Italian submarine. If Theresa worked through the supper hour, which she did often, more food was delivered to her by a restaurant courier service. Pasta was her favorite. Between these hurry-up meals, she drank coffee in the morning, switching to diet cola in the afternoon. "I know I need to watch my calories," she commented to me, taking a sip from a can of diet soda.

"Do you enjoy your meals?" I asked.

"They keep me going," she replied with a laugh.

I smiled. "So, what can I do for you?"

"I'm about thirty pounds overweight, and I need help to get it off in a hurry. There's a company-wide trip to Puerto Vallarta coming up in four months," she said. "My last trainer helped me a few years ago, but the weight came right back. I hate my body and how I look. I need something that will work for the long term, work fast, and I want to get started right away, so tell me what to do."

"This may be somewhat difficult for you, at least at first—"

She cut me off. "Don't worry about difficult," she said. "I can handle it."

"As I said," I continued. "It may be a challenge at first, but first we need to focus on learning to slow down and breathe."

"Slow down and breathe?" she shot back. "I don't think you understand. My day is organized in fifteen-minute increments. You see, I schedule everything in fifteen-minute time blocks. That's the only way I get things done. I don't have time to slow down and take it easy."

"Exactly my point," I said. "For most of us, we eat the way we do life. If we are in a hurry, rushed for time and anxious, we will hurriedly eat our meals. We may skip exercise, because we don't have the time. We need to slow down, breathe, and begin enjoying the pleasurable moments in life."

"Slow down? That makes no sense," she said. "If anything, I need more exercise. I need to do more, not less."

In the weeks that followed, I helped Theresa with food choices and an exercise routine that combined cardio with weight training. As she lost the weight, we talked about her slowing down to enjoy life's little pleasures, whether in the form of a tasty, nutritious meal, a son's soccer game, or a late evening bubble bath. To some extent, she slowed her maddening pace, and, by the time the Puerto Vallarta trip came around, she was swimsuit ready.

"Weight is the screen that prevents us from looking within for the whisper of who we truly are."
—*Ashly*

6:

Embrace Food, Embrace Life

When you eat a meal, do you taste the food? At first, that may seem a ridiculous question, but think about it. How often do you devour a meal, only to wonder, "Where did it go?" Perhaps you know it was good, but can you describe the taste of each item on the plate? Mindful eating is about being present at the moment you consume your food. Too often during a meal, we take a mindful vacation. Our minds are focused on conversation with family or friends, or a television program, or a news article, or a Facebook page, or any number of other distractions. Our eating goes into "autopilot mode," a series of chewing and swallowing motions with little or no actual enjoyment of the meal. In a sense, we shovel in the food to fill our belly for no other reason than the food is there to be shoveled.

The next time you sit down to a meal, become aware of the pleasures awaiting your palate, and taste a single bite. Relish the scent, flavors, and textures. Take it slow. Be deliberate. Be present. Enjoying meals mindfully takes practice, and, like sex, this kind of practice is fun, so bring your senses to the table. You can still converse during a meal. After all, few social activities are as rewarding as sharing a meal with others. Put down the fork, and share a thought. Then pick up the utensil and take another bite, again delighting in the scent, taste, and texture of the food in your mouth. Time and again, people who learn to eat mindfully notice they eat less.

In nearly all of us, there is a ravenous beast, a creature that devours the plate of food and is looking for more. Fortunately, usually as children, we learn to control the beast. However, for some, the beast is difficult to keep in check. A top athlete in high school and college, Melinda harbored dark, guilty secrets. Those who knew her best, family and friends, were proud of her achievements as a standout sprinter and hurdler: a First Team All-American in the 400-meter sprint, conference champion in the 60-meter hurdles, and her university's representative to the NCAA track and field championships. A high school coach turned her on to the benefits of carbohydrate loading, putting away large quantities of pastas and grains the night before a meet to fill the body with glycogen, the primary source of muscle energy. She continued the regimen when she earned a scholarship to run track at the university level.

The scholarship covered basic expenses, but each month Melinda came up short. A woman in the dorm told her about a job that earned good money, and the hours were always in the evening. That's how Melinda became an exotic dancer. At first, she was embarrassed to wrap herself around a pole and strip her clothes down to a barely visible G-string to the beat of thumping music and the hooting of the club's male patrons. Soon it became a guilty obsession. So as not to be recognized, she and her friend drove an hour to reach the club, located in an adjacent state, making it in time by skipping the dorm meal and eating fast food in the car.

A background of carbo loading, eating on the run, and the shame of being a stripper combined to become a perfect storm for a binge eater. Melinda told me nothing of this history when she sought my help a few months after graduation. "I want you to be my trainer and help keep me in shape," she said. "I'm starting graduate school in May at the University of Texas Southwestern Medical Center to get my degree as a physician's assistant."

We worked together for more than two years, becoming friends in the process. During that time, the former athlete, serious about her workouts, maintained a sculpted, muscled body that could have been featured on the cover of a fitness magazine. It was September, a month before Melinda was to graduate with her physician's assistant degree. "You're doing beautifully," I complimented her.

With a downcast demeanor and a note of sadness, she said, "I don't feel so beautiful. I feel ugly and dirty."

Astonished, I touched her shoulder. "Tell me what's troubling you," I asked tenderly. "Maybe I can help."

It was as if a bolt to a door locked long ago was suddenly released. Through tears and anguish, Melinda opened up to me about her private obsessions. Having been raised in a strict Christian home, she knew her second career as a stripper was a sin in the eyes of her parents and the church, but she found it exhilarating, a heart-pumping high stronger than winning any race on the track. Then, she told me about the excitement of fast food binge eating.

"There are times the anticipation of hitting the drive-through is a rush you can't believe," she explained. "You can't imagine how strong it is. It's like I'm another person. Something takes over. Funny thing, afterwards, I don't even remember doing it."

When the ravenous beast roared from deep within, Melinda typically drove to a Wendy's and ordered a triple hamburger with large fries, which she ate on the way to a McDonald's drive-thru, where she got a sack of fried chicken BLT sandwiches and more fries. The bag was empty by the time she steered to a Sonic for onion rings, mozzarella cheese sticks, and several chili cheese hotdogs. The road trip feast continued with a stop at Taco Bell for a bag of burritos and chalupas. The Taco Bell bags were empty, the car littered with food wrappers of all shapes and colors, when she pulled in behind a stream of cars at Dairy Queen for a large chocolate sundae and banana split. She'd consumed everything by the time she was back in her apartment.

"I'm so ashamed, Ashly," she cried. "I want to stop. I know what I'm doing is self-destructive, but I can't seem to do anything about it. Please help me."

For most of us, we are at times subject to some degree of obsessive-compulsive behavior. Maybe we worry too much, or check and re-check the door lock, drink too much, spend too much money, or shower several times a day to ward off illness. Ever "knock on wood" for luck? When a ritual-like compulsion becomes an obsession, a behavior that's out of control and possibly debilitating, professional intervention may be required.

The symptoms of obsessive-compulsive disorder (OCD), often appearing in the high school and college years, are usually the result of anxiety, brought on by academic challenges; the need to excel in sports; or difficult relationships with parents, siblings, or schoolmates. In adulthood, the stress of unemployment, marital issues, and childbirth can trigger OCD.

One of the most hidden obsessions in our society involves food, either the unleashing of the ravenous beast that takes over rational thought to devour everything in sight, or the rejection of nutrition altogether. Every year, men and women die from starvation, not because they can't get food, but because they refuse to eat, or, if they eat, they empty their stomach contents. The awareness of bulimia hit the headlines in 1983 when drummer and singer Karen Carpenter died at age thirty-two after subjecting herself to a water-only diet. Since then, the specter of bulimia arises every so often. To qualify for the U.S. Olympic team, gymnast Christy Henrich was told to lose weight. She did and died of multiple organ failure in 1994. She was twenty-two. Subsisting on a diet of only apples and tomatoes, Brazilian fashion model Ana Carolina Reston, who appeared in Giorgio Armani ads, died at age twenty-one.

At the opposite end of the eating disorder spectrum, overeating increases the risk of coronary heart disease, type 2 diabetes, certain cancers, high blood pressure, stroke, liver disease, osteoarthritis and sleep apnea. An indication of how much the obesity epidemic is changing the medical landscape is the sharp spike in sleep apnea cases. In the past twenty years, sleep apnea has increased 55 percent. All in all, medical care costs related to obesity in the United States top a staggering $150 billion.

Of all mental illnesses, eating disorders have the highest mortality rate. Among girls and women between the ages of fifteen and twenty-four, the mortality rate is twelve times higher than any other cause of death, including auto accidents and drug overdose. Only ten percent of individuals with eating disorders receive treatment.

Melinda made the decision to come out of the dark and seek help for her strip club exhibitionism and fast food binging. In working with individuals struggling with OCD eating disorders, I've learned not to confront the issue. It's not about controlling the compulsion or being vindictive and judgmental. The science is often debated, but in my experience, overeating is as much an addiction as alcohol or drugs, and, as such, requires understanding, empathy, and compassion. Unlike an addiction to alcohol or drugs, which are substances not essential to life, an addiction to food is much more difficult to kick, because nutrition is a requirement for living. Of note, many people who were once addicted to cigarettes later become addicted to food. They simply shift their addiction to another substance.

The healing process begins with acknowledging the addiction and realizing outside help is needed and progresses when the person understands why they have an addiction, forgives themselves for any wrongdoing to themselves or others, and makes a lifelong commitment to embrace a healthy lifestyle. Working with a psychologist, Melinda came to terms with her exhibitionism. Working together, we focused on her fast food compulsion.

Binging as well as overeating is not a lack of willpower. It's a lack of awareness. When we are aware of the food, taste it, take pleasure in it, and embrace it as the way to nourish ourselves, we are in the moment.

"When an overwhelming feeling of compulsion begins to overtake you, and you sense the ravenous beast is about to exert itself, take a deep breath and become aware of the moment," I taught Melinda. "A compulsion, such as fast food binging, cannot coexist with awareness. It's impossible. A compulsive act cannot take place in a mindful moment."

Then I gave Melinda an assignment. Initially she was skeptical, but after two more episodes of fast food binging, she tried it. Here was the assignment: Instead of immediately devouring each bag of fast food, place the bags in the back seat. Take them home and go through the ritual of preparing an elegant feast complete with your finest china, table linen, goblet, and place setting. Put on your favorite music and turn the lights down low. Light a candle and open each sack, deliberately positioning every item on the plates. If you wish to begin with the Wendy's triple hamburger, go right ahead, but be sure to take your time, taste each and every morsel, savor the flavor, and relish the meal. Turn your attention to the McDonald's fried chicken BLT sandwich. Be aware of the sandwich. Delight in the aroma, experience the crispy fried texture, and enjoy it to the fullest. Continue your mindful banquet with the Sonic onion rings, mozzarella cheese sticks, and chili cheese hotdogs. Stay in the moment and take pleasure in the Taco Bell burritos and chalupas. Finally, finish the meal with the Dairy Queen chocolate sundae and banana split.

At our next session, I asked, "How did it go? Did you enjoy your banquet?"

"At first, I was doubtful this approach would work, but I did what you recommended, and, to my amazement, the ravenous beast we've talked about never appeared," Melinda reported. "I was able to eat some of the hamburger and a little of the chicken sandwich. By the time I got to the onion rings, I was getting pretty full. I stopped after one cheese stick. I was stuffed. I couldn't believe that many times I have been able to eat all that stuff and have room for the DQ."

"That's because you stayed in the moment," I said, congratulating her on the breakthrough. "When we are mindful and aware of what we are doing, it's impossible to be compulsive."

Apply awareness to overcome the ravenous beast. I call this technique "Formalizing the Binge." It takes practice, so be patient with yourself, because the more you formalize the binge, the more aware you will become and the less you will depend on the beast. That's because we invent the monster as a form of protection, something that shields us from fears, hurts, shame, and painful emotions. The beast prevents us from facing and dealing with realities. When it is about to emerge, repeat this brief statement:

"Hello, Ravenous Beast, I know you are here to protect me, but I have become strong and sure. I no longer need your protection. I thank you for standing up for me when I needed you, but I don't need you now. You can take a rest. I am in charge of my life. I'm embracing every aspect of who I am."

Here are steps you can take to formalize the binge:

- At the moment you are feeling the ravenous beast is about to be released, acknowledge it. Be aware and present with it. Take time to breathe, relax, and become mindful.
- Decide which foods you want, prepare them, or get them.
- Create a beautiful meal setting by using your best china, light candles, and put on soothing music.
- Take a moment to be grateful for the meal.
- Look at the plate of foods you love and crave. Be present in the moment.
- Bring your senses to life. Be mindful of the food's appearance, aroma, and the ambiance of the meal.

- Gradually, and with intention, taste the first bite. Take in all the flavors and textures. Chew the food and enjoy every ounce. Swallow and feel the food enter your body.
- Take a second bite. Commune with the food. Slow your eating to a leisurely pace. If the ravenous beast makes an appearance, talk to the beast. Let the beast know you are in control of the meal.
- As thoughts and fears surface, allow them to breathe, and come up for air. Acknowledge these thoughts and release them.
- Slowly continue to enjoy every nuance of the meal.
- Finally, take note of all that transpired. You will realize that in this relaxed state of dining, you tamed the ravenous beast. You confronted the emotions, fears, shame, or whatever controlled you, freed yourself, and restored a sense of peace and tranquility within.

Embrace the food that nourishes your body, and you are embracing life.

"It is vitally important to be healthy and self-approved versus thin and fittin' in."
—Ashly

7:

Who's Coming to Dinner?

You are about to eat, a napkin is in your lap, and food is on your plate. It may be enlightening to check in before biting in. Ask yourself, "Who is coming to dinner?" Depending on your mood, the pressures of the day, your outlook on life, any number of personas may be seated at your place at mealtime.

The princess who demands, "By golly, this is what I want, and I want it now."

The stubborn, bratty child who shrieks, "I'm not eating this gross stuff."

The king: "I'm eating anything and everything I want, because I'm the king."

Or, are you showing up at mealtimes as the empowered adult responsible for your actions? This is the individual who says, "I will eat healthful portions of vegetables, fruits, grains, dairy, and protein. I will eat to make sure my body functions at peak performance, so I can fulfill my purpose. Nothing more. Nothing less."

Too often, we let the events of our day determine the person who arrives at mealtimes and sits in our chair. The stimulus may be an upsetting conversation with a supervisor or co-worker. Possibly you received a stressful phone call from a family member. There could be worries about money, a concern about a child's behavior, a fight with a spouse, or an argument with a neighbor. When we are upset or anxious, our minds are somewhere else. We're certainly not thinking about the meal we are about to consume.

For Delia, food was an escape. In the eyes of her husband and children, she never did anything right. It wasn't always this way. In college, while earning a degree in marketing, she was an officer in her sorority, a member of the glee club, and worked on the student newspaper. When meeting Blake at a Greek Week event, Delia was a petite blonde with a winning smile. Their romance immediately warmed, and, following graduation, they married in the college Georgian chapel. Flash forward fifteen years. With three boys between the ages of nine and fourteen, Delia worked about eighteen hours a week at a women's boutique. Blake was in television advertising sales.

"At the boutique, I do okay," Delia told me. "At home, no matter what I do, it's never up to par. The house is not orderly enough. Blake's favorite shirt has not been cleaned and pressed. I don't do things the way Blake thinks they should be done, and he lets me know it in no uncertain terms. The kids are the same way. All I hear, all day long, is criticism."

"For example, what happened recently that made you think you did not do something right?" I asked.

"Okay, on Saturday, while everyone was away at a ball game, I decided to wash Blake's SUV as a surprise. I scrubbed and cleaned the car inside and out, and I thought it looked great," she related. "When Blake saw it, he told me I didn't rinse the soap off the right way, and so there were streaks. He took it to the carwash."

"How did that make you feel?"

"Like a failure."

Little wonder that at mealtimes, Delia was beaten, rejected, and feeling inadequate. She took solace in food, silently gulping down her meal as Blake and the children talked about their day, sports, or television. Poor eating habits contributed to her weight gain, furthering the inferiority complex.

Coming to me for help to lose the excess weight, Delia needed to see for herself who was dining in her chair at mealtimes; not the capable adult that she was, but an alter-ego filled with self-defeating beliefs. Over the years, Delia had internalized feelings of inadequacy to the point that she was convinced her husband, children, and just about everyone else in her life were superior. She needed to replace inferiority with confidence. Delia, like each of us, was placed on this earth with a purpose and outfitted with the talents and gifts to fulfill that purpose. She needed to discern that direction.

In addition to coaching her about food choices and developing an exercise routine she could follow, I suggested Delia commit her thoughts to a journal. Journaling helps clients see themselves in a different, more objective light. The act of placing one's thoughts and feelings on paper often helps address emotional conflicts and suggests insights into self-destructive behavior.

Over the next several months, Delia faithfully described her private thoughts in the journal. With her permission, we read them together before each of our workouts, and, for the first time in her life, she became introspective about her dreams, needs, and wants. Using her marketing background, she became a volunteer at a large children's hospital, assisting with a fund-raising campaign. Food became a means to having the health and vitality she wanted for her body, and no longer served as an escape from unhappiness. As she gained confidence, her marriage improved and so did the relationships with her children. She had a new sense of the role she was meant to play in the world. Most recently, the hospital's development office created a staff position for her. She calls on individual and corporate donors and has generated a number of substantial cash gifts for the institution.

The following are life-affirming acts all of us can add to our daily activities to enrich our lives:

- Awake with a smile, and consider five blessings in your life.
- Breathe deeply. Imagine you are absorbing joy, peace, serenity, and love.
- In the mirror, affirm you are capable, gifted, and talented. Say to yourself, "I rock!" and mean it.
- Select outfits that reflect your style and optimism.
- Spend time with those who affirm and build you up.
- Set aside time each day for quiet reflection.
- Encourage others and offer help where needed.
- Be yourself and enjoy your best life.
- End the day with thoughts of gratitude.

When it came to relationships, Adrienne attracted abusive men like a magnet. The only girl in a family of four boys, she had been belittled and badgered for as far back as she could remember. Her mother died of cancer when she was in middle school. After that, her father criticized her for not being smart enough, not being thin enough, or pretty enough. Following their dad's lead, her brothers teased and taunted her to tears. As a high school senior, to get away from her family, she got pregnant, had a quick wedding, and moved to Texas with her new husband, an auto mechanic. The abuse continued at the hands of her volatile spouse until he was incarcerated for beating a fellow employee with a tire iron. The divorce was nearly as quick as the wedding. Two abusive boyfriends later, Adrienne was psychologically battered, emotionally bruised, and at the mercy of her ravenous beast.

At one of our first sessions, I asked, "When are you the happiest, Adrienne?"

"Do you want the truth?"

"If you want to tell me the truth, I'm here to listen," I said.

"I'm happy when I eat," she matter-of-factly stated.

"Anything else?"

"Not really. I live for food."

Like many people, Adrienne lived to eat rather than ate to live.

That's tragic, because our world offers so much more to enjoy besides taking comfort in our next meal. Life is not meant to be tolerated and endured. It's meant to be celebrated with a large measure of passion, fulfillment, and pleasure. A joy-filled life is a happy life, and we all deserve that.

When we enjoy pleasurable moments that are not food related, we still heat up our metabolism. It's a fact; when a person experiences joy, the body naturally produces endorphins in the brain as well as in the digestive system. In the biochemistry of our bodies, endorphins are the molecules of pleasure, existing to make us happy, but that's not all. Endorphins play a role in helping us burn fat. That means the happier we are, the more fat we burn.

Research teams at Oxford University and at the Montreal Neurological Institute at McGill University have tracked how the brain's centers for emotions and rewards respond to pleasurable activities. A kind of euphoria results from food, sex, music, and any number of activities that would be considered pleasurable. According to the human brain studies, if we fail to experience healthy pleasures on a day-to-day basis, we become restless and anxious. The absence of pleasure leads to increased levels of stress.

The answer to having more happiness? Seek pleasurable moments. Pet a dog, get a body massage, listen to a symphony, join in a lively discussion, stroll through an art museum, or do whatever else you find pleasurable. Which activities can help you pass the time? Planting and tending a garden, a round of golf, playing a musical instrument, or reading a book are a few that fall into this category.

Suggesting Adrienne consider pleasures that are not food-related, I proposed making a "gusto list." Instead of food, what could she do to help her feel happy, satisfied, content, and live life with gusto? To stimulate her thinking, I came up with a series of "gusto list" questions:

- What makes you smile?
- What makes you laugh and feel good?
- At what times during your day are you the happiest?
- In the past few weeks, what experiences did you find pleasurable?
- What brings you the most satisfaction?
- When do you feel content?

As a result of making the list, we determined Adrienne enjoyed her morning shower and beautifying herself for the day, but, in the rush of her life, seldom took time for these simple pleasures. The norm was a quick shower and throwing on a little blush.

"We need to slow things down," I suggested with a smile. "Let's make your morning a pleasurable ritual." Going to bed an hour earlier, Adrienne gave herself the pleasure of an hour each morning, just for herself, consisting of a leisurely shower and time to apply makeup. It was the beginning of Adrienne's healing and transformation from feeling like a victim to feeling empowered. She learned to appreciate and embrace her body as the exceptional temple that it was, and she gave herself permission to seek pleasure in the everyday occurrences happening all around her. Adrienne slowed down at mealtimes, too, savoring the aromas, tastes, and textures of the food. She nourished her body, so she could enjoy life's abundant pleasures.

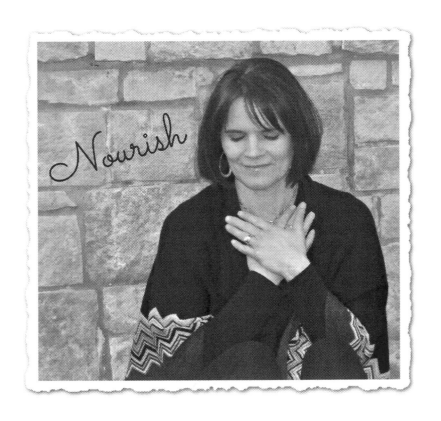

PART 2

weight problems, whether a person is underweight or overweight based on height and age as compared to the overall population.

According to the BMI, I carry about ten pounds more than what is considered average. At the so-called average weight for a woman of my height and age, I'm not at my best. I feel weak, lethargic, and not mentally sharp. My "natural" weight is perfect for me, and my overall level of fitness permits me to fulfill my life purposes, which include my work as a personal trainer. What is your natural weight? That depends much more on your purpose than the BMI screening tool.

This is the question we should ask: What is your ideal level of fitness? Fitness speaks to the foods we eat, the amount of activity our bodies require, and the wholesomeness of our thoughts. We are responsible for nourishing all three.

At times, a new client, learning about the **END Zone** philosophy, will inquire, "Does this mean you are giving me permission to eat anything I desire, and it's not a big deal?" No, because the foods we consume are definitely a "big deal." That's why it's best to eat according to your life purpose. Similar to the concept of "shapeshifting," the reshaping of our attitudes and beliefs in the image of the person we want to be requires we eat like the person we want to become.

Selected to participate in a television reality game show that brought together a number of single men to compete for the hand of a young woman, Martin wanted to get in shape. "Help me get the ripped body of a movie star," he told me. "I've got to be lean and muscular, with six-pack abs like that guy on *Hawaii Five-0*, because I want to look amazing in the hot tub scene."

"You're talking about Alex O'Loughlin?"

"Yep, that's the guy," he replied enthusiastically. "I want to be that guy."

With that image in mind, we went to work on Martin's food choices, meals containing protein and vegetables and no complex carbohydrates, such as whole grains that require longer periods to digest. Simultaneously, he adopted an intensive weight training regimen. Losing twenty pounds and gaining a film-star physique, Martin was a knockout in the show's hot tub. He didn't win the girl, but when he ran into a woman he had known in high school, she was impressed. "You look fantastic!" she exclaimed. They are now married, and I became her trainer as well.

"Shapeshifting" to become whom you want to be is not always as dramatic as Martin's story, but if you set your mind on living a particular way, everything seems to fall into place, and your life develops accordingly. About every year, the girls in my family, Mom, my sisters and sisters-in-law, plan a brief getaway just for us. For one of our girls-only vacations, we rented a condo on a beach in Maui. I wanted to look good in my bikini, but I was feeling "fluffy." My pants were snug, and I knew I'd gained some extra pounds. Looking in the mirror, instead of seeing the fluffiness around my middle, I imagined my body as I wanted it to appear. I began repeating this mantra, "I am beautiful in my bikini." Almost immediately, I began eating in alignment with the image I wanted for myself. I ate smaller portions and chose foods that digested well without leaving me bloated. Repeating the mantra often, I selected foods that supported the look I wanted. The fluffiness was replaced with lean muscle in time for the flight to Hawaii. I was beautiful in my bikini.

Most of us are all too familiar with the types of foods that are counterproductive to helping us be as fit as we need to be, such as layer cakes, cream pies, doughnuts, and the other incredibly tasty treats that our figurative sweet tooth craves, but what are the productive kinds of foods we should consider? As a rule-of-thumb, fresh is best. Whenever practical, rely on fresh rather than canned, frozen, or freeze-dried, because you can be better assured the nutritional contents of the foods are of the highest possible value. Research shows that most varieties of vegetables lose substantial levels of vitamins within days of harvesting. Since we do not know how long vegetables were in cold storage before processing, the nutritional content at the time of canning is a mystery. We do know the heating process of canning vegetables destroys as much as half of the vitamin A, vitamin C, thiamin, and riboflavin.

While fresh vegetables and fruits are best, frozen is a good choice in the "off-season," when fresh can be expensive or is not available. Before flash-freezing, vegetables are blanched in hot water or with steam, which tends to break down nutrients such as vitamin C and vitamin B. The freeze-drying of foods depletes to a degree most nutrients, including vitamin C, vitamin E, and folic acid.

Another rule-of-thumb: Buy organic. It's not always possible to purchase organic foods due to availability and price, but the difference can be significant. Conventionally grown foods are subject to chemical fertilizers meant to promote faster and thicker growth and are sprayed with synthetic insecticides. Synthetic herbicides are used to control weeds. In terms of cattle, swine, chickens, and other animals, growth hormones, antibiotics and other medications are mega-farm staples. On the other side of the fence, organic farmers feed soil and plants with manure or compost, use naturally derived sprays, count on beneficial insects and birds as part of the growing process, and feed the animals with organic foods. Animals are usually given access to outdoor ranges to minimize the spread of diseases. In one study, nearly a quarter of farms with caged hens tested positive for salmonella compared to 4.4 percent in organic flocks. Another important difference is that organic farmers do not use genetically modified seed, a recent agricultural development with unknown long-term health implications.

We know a balanced diet contains complex carbohydrates such as fruits and vegetables, protein, and fat. However, many people are confused about portion size, specifically how much of any one of these is appropriate. Here's another rule-of-thumb: The size of your hand is the amount of complex carbs you need; make a fist and that's the amount of protein; the size of your thumb is the fat.

Deb was a year away from her tenth wedding anniversary. "When Jack and I married, we wanted to bicycle through northern Europe," she told me, wistfully describing the sights they would have visited such as the ancient city of Bruges, the tulip fields and windmills of Holland, and Northern Germany's Schwerin Castle. "Graduate school got in the way, but we've made the decision to turn back the clock. Next year, for our anniversary, we're biking on the continent."

"Wonderful," I said. "Congratulations. How can I help?"

"I guess age is catching up with me," she responded with a joyful laugh. "I need to get in shape, if I'm pedaling in Europe next summer, and that means getting back to my bridal weight. I need to lose about thirty pounds."

Willing to change her eating habits, Deb imagined the shape she would be in when the June anniversary came around, and I suggested she keep a "food log," a notebook to track the foods she ate. Unfailingly, Deb recorded every morsel she placed in her mouth while eating slowly and mindfully.

"I'm surprised how much food I ate before I really took notice of my eating habits," she remarked at one of our weekly sessions. "I'm not snacking like I once did," she continued. "I'm eating healthier foods and in smaller portions, but I'm not hungry."

As the weight came off, Deb bicycled on weekend trips with her husband as a way to strengthen her legs and build endurance. Over the year, she lost a total of thirty-five pounds. Returning from the bike trip in Belgium, The Netherlands, and Germany, she proudly showed me photos of herself with Jack at Schwerin, often referred to as Cinderella's castle. With the intent to keep biking, she has remained Cinderella-trim for a number of years. One of Deb's purposes in life is to accompany her husband on the bike trips they love.

"Weight loss is really about living at your natural weight in a fun, pleasurable, love-filled way."
—Ashly

9:

Purge the Pantry

Processed foods are a primary contributor to America's obesity challenge. According to the University of Washington's Center for Public Health Nutrition, affordable and convenient processed foods, such as ready-to-eat breakfast cereals, pancake mixes, crackers, pizza dough, tortilla shells, noodles, spaghetti, and macaroni, made with refined grains, added sugars, and supplemented with fats for taste, contribute to the overweight condition of the population. Refined grains, also known as flours, the basis for a huge assortment of processed foods, become sugar in the body. "Refined carbohydrates, including refined grain products, are the single most harmful influence in the American diet today," states Dr. David Ludwig, director of the New Balance Foundation Obesity Prevention Center at Children's Hospital Boston.

Foods made with refined grains enter the body and are absorbed into the bloodstream as simple sugars. Blood-sugar levels quickly spike, and, just as quickly, crash. As a result, you feel tired, sleepy, and lethargic. As the body reacts, these foods trigger sugar and carbohydrate cravings so overwhelming we can't get enough of them. When the marketers issue the challenge, "Can't eat just one," they're spot on. Purge your pantry, refrigerator, and acids and polyphenols such as olive oil. Also consider coconut oil, grapeseed oil, and flaxseed oil.

Rather than baking with all-purpose bleached flour, use high-protein grain, like quinoa seed, which offers essential amino acids such as lysine and lots of calcium, iron, and phosphorus. Cooked much like rice, quinoa seed is available in a flour form for making pancakes and baking bread.

Hemp, whey, or rice protein powders are good to have on hand to mix in fruit smoothies.

Stock up on zucchini, yellow squash, spaghetti squash, butternut squash, acorn squash, beets, sweet potatoes, white potatoes, avocados, coconut, bananas, pears, and apples. Select beans such as dried lentils, as well as black, pinto, kidney, and garbanzo.

Rely on fresh vegetables of all kinds. Consider green beans, carrots, celery, portabella mushrooms, spinach, romaine, collard greens, kale, chard, grape tomatoes, and olives. Also buy fruits such as cherries and grapes.

In the meats area, purchase chicken breast, white fish, salmon, lamb, beef, ostrich, and pork tenderloin.

An alternative to dairy, hemp milk is an excellent choice of protein and contains ten essential amino acids. Other nondairy substitutes include coconut milk, rich in medium-chain fatty acids, thought to promote weight maintenance; almond milk, which contains no cholesterol or lactose; and rice milk. In terms of cheese, look for parmesan (not the processed cheese powder), goat, feta, and sheep cheeses.

Season your food with Himalayan sea salt and fresh herbs, such as rosemary, thyme, and sage. Sweeten with blackstrap molasses, an excellent source of vitamin B6, calcium, magnesium, iron, and potassium; stevia, an outstanding sugar substitute that has little effect on blood glucose; and raw honey.

Use tortillas made from freshly sprouted, organic whole kernel corn or whole grain. Sprouted grains are easier to digest than processed flour and contain antioxidants and increased levels of vitamin C and vitamin B.

When it comes to nuts, stay away from salted nuts and nuts roasted in hydrogenated oils or saturated fats. Instead, select raw, unsalted nuts. The healthiest nuts include almonds, cashews, peanuts, and walnuts. Pumpkin seeds, sesame seeds, sunflower seeds, and flaxseeds offer a number of nutritional benefits.

Enjoy the journey to healthier eating. Take it one step at a time, experiment with recipes, and have fun discovering new tastes and better ways to nourish your body.

Spice, today known as Victoria Beckham, was photographed with a copy of the *Skinny Bitch* diet book in 2007, women and men became vegetarians by the droves, limiting their foods to mainly fruits and vegetables. Dr. Barry Sears instructed adherents of his "Zone Diet" to regulate their body's insulin production and balance hormones. There will always be diets du jour, and, just as certainly, adherents will lose weight, at least in the short term.

Since we all have different physiology and nutritional requirements, we each need to determine the foods and portions that are best for us. Experiment by making three lists: the foods you enjoy the most; the healthy foods you believe would be beneficial for your lifestyle; and, finally, the special foods you consider treats. One of my clients, Rob, the owner and CEO of a real estate development company, told me he had tried nearly every diet under the sun, but all failed to keep him trim year after year. "Most recently, I was a vegetarian for a year, but I felt weak and had bouts of lightheadedness," he related. "I went back to eating meat. As if making up for lost time, I can't get enough of it. I crave beef, chicken, any meat, but I know I shouldn't be eating that much of it."

Not surprisingly, on Rob's list of "Foods I Enjoy Most," beef was first, followed by chicken and meatloaf. To the list, he added salmon, lobster tail, crab cakes, western omelet, steak fajitas, tortilla soup, clam chowder, Reuben sandwiches, and anything barbecued.

On the "healthy foods" list he specified apples, oranges, bananas, broccoli, cauliflower, squash, wild rice, sweet potatoes, and eggplant.

Listed as "special treats" were key lime pie, roasted peanuts, potato chips, pizza, fried chicken, and chocolate chip cookies, especially when served warm with ice cream.

Open to suggestions, Rob worked with me to expand the "healthy foods" choices with the addition of tomatoes, steel-cut oatmeal, quinoa, bulgur, flaxseeds, almonds, full-fat Greek yogurt, Brussels sprouts, red beets, lentils, kidney beans, spinach, blueberries, pumpkin, walnuts, and kale.

"We want you to eat healthy and balanced meals, but that doesn't mean cutting out all the foods you like best," I counseled. "Our goal is to have you eating eighty percent wholesome good-for-you foods and the balance, the twenty percent, the fluff, meaning the foods you love such as that key lime pie or warm chocolate chip cookies with ice cream."

Over a period of about three months, we gradually altered Rob's eating habits by progressively introducing healthier foods while reducing the less beneficial options. At first, the balance between healthy foods and "fluff" was roughly fifty-fifty. By the end of the third month, the real estate developer was on his way to an eighty-twenty dietary menu. That didn't mean Rob could not have chips and salsa one night or an occasional pepperoni and sausage pizza, but his consumption of nourishing foods improved dramatically. With moderate aerobic exercise and twice-a-week muscle-building activity, Rob's weight and general state of health aligned with his needs. Since it was a measured process without drastic dieting, he said it felt natural and easy. We changed Rob's mindset about the foods he ate, and, in so doing, placed him on the road to a longer and healthier life.

Whether you're an athlete in training or someone like Rob, working to advance your business or career, I offer six basic fitness regimens that benefit every lifestyle:

Drink twelve cups of water a day. Unable to store water, the body requires ample fresh water every day. As much as seventy-five percent of our body is made up of water, and water is essential for every bodily function, as minute as what happens in individual cells to the operation of every organ and overall blood flow. In fact, blood is ninety percent water. For that reason, when we do not drink enough water, the body goes searching for it, and one of the initial sources is the water in the bloodstream. As the body pulls water from the blood, the blood becomes thicker, more difficult to pump, and is at risk of clotting. Lack of adequate water is thought to contribute to hypertension, concentrated levels of cholesterol in the blood, and heart disease. Frequent headaches and bouts of heartburn may be linked to a lack of sufficient water. We can survive several days without food, but we will soon perish without water.

- Go easy on bread and foods made with grains, particularly refined grains such as white flour. When consuming grains, eat them earlier in the day, no later than 2 p.m., because the body breaks them down into glucose as an instant form of energy. Unless you worked off the glucose before bedtime, that pasta dinner was stored in the fat cells. Eating grains sparingly lowers blood pressure, reduces the risk of diabetes, and helps get rid of abdominal fat.

- Before downing foods from the twenty percent "fluff" list (think Rob's warm chocolate chip cookie topped with ice cream), ask yourself three questions, but be honest. Am I truly hungry for this treat? Will this contribute to body muscle or fat? Do I really need to have this? It's not so much about taking yourself on a guilt trip for splurging on unhealthy food choices, but more about mindfully attending to your body's physiological needs on your journey through life.

- To help make smarter food selections, measure the "fluff" choice from the list of exceptions against the most delicious exception food you can imagine. Does it measure up? You are at a birthday party. The hostess offers you a gaily decorated paper plate covered with triple chocolate cake and two scoops of moose tracks ice cream. Does this birthday treat match or exceed the tastiest delicacy you can conjure up? If not, politely decline. Save your twenty percent quota of fluff foods for the goodies you actually want to eat.

- Take your body out for some exercise at least forty minutes a day, five days a week. On two of those days, concentrate on aerobic activities such as yoga or some other form of fun movement. Perhaps you enjoy swimming, dancing, tennis, or working in the garden. Aerobic activities that increase breathing and heart rate keep the lungs, heart, and circulatory system strong and healthy. On the other three days of the week, treat your body to resistance and high intensity training. According to a recent study, only one in five Americans exercises enough to keep the body physically fit. Guidelines issued by the U.S. Department of Health recommend at least 150 minutes a week (30 minutes, 5 days a week) of moderate aerobic exercise plus muscle-building activity twice a week.
- Think good thoughts. Empower yourself by having a positive thought life. Upbeat and optimistic people are more likely to handle stress better and be healthier in mind, body, and spirit. Keeping a positive attitude does not imply ignoring the unhappiness in our world. It's about taking a proactive and productive approach. On the whole, individuals who are positive and optimistic eat healthier, exercise more, refrain from excessively drinking alcoholic beverages, and do not smoke. As a result, they live longer. Consider positive thoughts such as: "I am healthy and strong," "I make wise food choices," "I am joyfully and wonderfully made," and "I am enough."

In addition to the six basic fitness regimens, clients often inquire about meal plans. Similar to food choices, meal plans are subject to personal preference. The basic daily meal plan that works for me is comprised of one main meal at lunchtime; two mini meals, one at breakfast and the other at the traditional dinner hour; and one to two snacks throughout the day.

I begin the morning with a "mini meal" breakfast of one portion of lean protein, one portion of fruits or vegetables, and one essential fat such as olives or olive oil, avocado, fresh coconut or coconut oil, nuts or seeds. A favorite breakfast consists of plain Greek yogurt, high in protein and low in sugar; oatmeal, a concentrated source of nutrients and fiber; fresh or frozen berries; and three tablespoons of fresh coconut sprinkled on the oatmeal.

A midmorning snack can be a serving of fruit, or a serving of vegetables, or nuts, or seeds. I enjoy an apple or fifteen almonds.

The noontime "main meal" includes a protein, two vegetable portions, one essential fat, and a whole grain, if desired.

A mid-afternoon snack can again be a serving of fruit, or a serving of vegetables, or nuts, or seeds.

The evening dinner hour "mini meal" is made up of one lean protein, one vegetable, and an essential fat.

At times, I substitute a smoothie for a meal. Thought to have originated in Brazil, the milkshake-like smoothie has become a healthy staple throughout the world. It's easy, convenient, tasty, and contains many of the nutritional benefits required by our active bodies. In addition to the hundreds of smoothie recipes available online, experiment with foods and tastes you enjoy. In a blender, toss in favorite fruits, vegetables, and additives such as flaxseeds, cocoa, coconut, or vanilla. Many people enhance their smoothies with honey, soy milk, green tea, and whey, hemp, rice, or another protein powder. When a smoothie is rich in vitamins, minerals, and fiber, it can play a big part in maintaining health, vigor, and fitness.

Eat foods in order to enjoy living your best life. Eat in moderation, acknowledging the importance of foods that supply the energy and strength to perform at your peak, and slow down to relish the infinite spectrum of tastes, textures, and delights available from our planet's land, sea, and sky.

"Make an appointment with your muscles, and then keep it."
—Ashly

11:

Muscles; Use Them or Lose Them

Nourishment involves more than the foods and beverages we consume. We nourish our bodies with exercise and movement, essential to keeping us physiologically whole and productive. Case in point: After a severe automobile accident, a fifty-five-year-old woman, unconscious and confined to a hospital bed, began losing muscle strength within a week. Two months after the accident, she came out of a coma, but was unable to raise her arms or move her legs. To regain muscle strength, doctors said four days of therapy were required for every day in bed. Subsequently, eight months of physical therapy and rehabilitation were required before the woman was strong enough to leave the hospital. Muscle atrophy is rapid and immediate. That's why astronauts at the International Space Station regularly exercise and condition muscles. Failure to do so would leave them powerless in earth gravity.

Just as muscles will atrophy from misuse, over time, they can also be strengthened and toned. That's the good news for individuals who have been living a relatively sedentary lifestyle such as office workers or anyone seated at a desk most of the day. Just as in the case of the fifty-five-year-old accident victim, therapy must start gradually, beginning with the use of resistance bands to gain strength before proceeding to more intense exercise routines.

Benefiting every aspect of our lives, exercise and physical activity deter diseases such as diabetes, coronary afflictions, breast and colon cancer, and osteoporosis; improve our ability to think and reason; boost feelings of confidence and general wellbeing; and give us the strength to do what we want to do.

There are basically four types of exercise and physical activity: endurance, strength, balance, and flexibility. Nourishing our bodies requires all four, and some activities fit into more than one of these categories. For instance, an endurance activity, such as running, builds strength. Bicycling, a strength activity, enhances balance.

Endurance activities fall into the aerobics field of fitness. Power walking, jogging, running, swimming and biking increase our breathing, jump our heart rate, and recharge the circulatory system. These are the activities that get the blood moving. A game of basketball, a tennis match, rowing a boat, and shoveling snow all build endurance.

Strength training builds muscle capacity. By using resistance bands, weights, and machines, we develop the back, chest, abs, shoulders, arms, and legs. As the muscles gain strength, we can progress to more challenging workouts.

Tai chi and yoga offer excellent routines to improve overall balance, coordination, range of motion, and posture. Defined as the intricate interrelationship of mind and body, balance enhances performance while reducing the risk of injury.

Flexibility exercises stretch the muscles to make the body more limber and agile. For the beginner, flexibility routines are a good place to start and can be accomplished in an office setting. Sitting in a work station, with a computer and keyboard at the ready, mouse in-hand, can be debilitating. Poor posture and a deskbound existence often contribute to severe back pain, tension headaches, and a general lack of blood circulation. A few times a day, take a moment to stretch. While seated, roll the shoulders. Start by making small circles and work up to make larger ones.

Roll the shoulders in a forward direction ten times. Roll them in the reverse direction ten times. While still seated in the chair, pull in the abs while leaning over and placing the hands on the floor in front of you. Hold for fifteen seconds. Repeat three times. Seated on the floor, press the feet together, pull in on the abs, and lean forward until you feel the hamstring muscles begin to stretch. Hold for fifteen seconds then relax. Repeat three times. Here's another: Take a lunge position by placing a knee on the floor. Position the opposite leg in a ninety-degree angle. Pull in the abs and press the hips forward, feeling the muscles on the front leg and hip area stretch. Hold for fifteen seconds and repeat three times. Change legs and do it again.

We typically schedule times for meals. Movement and exercise deserve no less attention. For example, just as you set aside thirty minutes for a lunch break, take a thirty-minute exercise break. Think of this time as a business appointment with yourself, and who is more important to your health than you? As important as a doctor's appointment, your daily exercise appointment is critical to your long-term health. Do not break it. Do not sleep through it. Honor it, because you honor and value your body.

Calisthenics, introduced by the military to shape up soldiers for duty, became a mainstream phenomenon in the early days of television when a San Francisco fitness instructor, Jack LaLanne, urged homemakers to get off the couch and join him for a round of jumping jacks, but LaLanne wasn't always so athletic. An overweight teenager surviving on junk food and candy, Jack was a hot-tempered high school dropout suffering from severe headaches. Hearing a lecture about nutrition and fitness, the fifteen-year-old started daily workouts, changed his eating habits, and turned his life around, going back to high school and attending college. Today, health and fitness clubs are everywhere, but Jack opened the nation's first, becoming a pioneer in the fitness movement in 1936. Immediately, his club in Oakland, California came under fire from local physicians who erroneously warned their patients that working out with weights would make them "muscle-bound," sap the sex drive, and cause heart attacks. Undeterred, Jack kept the club open, won converts, and went on to invent the leg-extension and cable and pulley weight machines that are now in every fitness club in the world.

In 1954, to promote his local fitness show on San Francisco TV, Jack LaLanne swam the length of the Golden Gate Bridge, nine-thousand feet, underwater with 140 pounds of air tanks and gear strapped to his back. It was a world record that still stands. He was forty years old. Going nationwide on ABC in 1959, LaLanne introduced his fitness show by performing a thousand jumping jacks and a thousand chin-ups in less than ninety minutes. Jack's exercise broadcasts were an ABC staple, remaining on the air until 1985. Proving that fitness can be a lifelong pursuit, at the age of seventy, Jack LaLanne, handcuffed and shackled, towed a string of seventy rowboats through heavy currents the one mile from Long Beach Harbor's Queen's Way Bridge to the Queen Mary.

LaLanne favored weight training and calisthenics, lunges, crunches, jumping jacks, sit-ups, pushups, and the like, to strengthen major muscle groups; however, the concept of endurance-based aerobic exercise is a relatively new development. A former Air Force colonel, Dr. Kenneth H. Cooper, inventing "aerobics" in 1968 with the publication of a book on the subject, went on to operate a chain of aerobics fitness centers in Texas. Seemingly overnight, aerobics moves were set to music, and dance exercise was an immediate hit. One of the earliest proponents of dance aerobics was Judi Sheppard Missett, launching Jazzercise franchises in 1969. Teaching jazz moves in a Chicago dance school, Judi started "just for fun" classes. The students loved it, and, soon, Judi was training Jazzercise instructors seemingly everywhere. Today, an estimated thirty-thousand Jazzercise classes take place every week throughout the U.S. and in more than thirty other nations.

Down in Colombia, Beto Perez, an aerobics dance instructor,

arriving to lead a class, discovered he left his jazz music at home. With no time to fetch the music he always used, Beto had to improvise, so, rooting through his backpack, he came up with several favorite salsas and merengue music tapes. Popping in one of the tapes, he started the class. Zumba was born. The Colombia sensation, coming to the U.S. in 2001 when Beto and two friends introduced a series of Zumba home videos, rapidly spread around the world. An estimated fourteen million people exercise to Zumba samba and mambo dance moves in nearly every corner of the earth.

By combining Jack LaLanne-style weight training, often called anaerobic exercise, and Zumba-like aerobics, you are burning fat and building muscle. The difference between anaerobic exercise and aerobics boils down to how various muscles burn energy and for how long. The foods we consume, whether protein, carbs, or fat, are turned into a chemical called adenosine triphosphate (ATP), which is the only chemical our body can burn for energy. Biologists consider ATP to be the energy currency of life, because it acts much like the contents of a battery, powering the functions that keep us alive, and then recharging by taking in the energy from glucose, which is derived from the foods we eat. When we breathe, the oxygen that fills our lungs travels to every cell in the body, and, at the cellular level, interacts with glucose to make ATP. By taking in huge gulps of oxygen during long-lasting aerobic exercise, we convert more food (glucose) to make the ATP that's burned to power our pumping arms, legs, and other muscles. That's what is meant by burning calories.

After we eat a meal, the food that is digested is turned into the glucose that energizes the ATP that powers our bodies for about eight to twelve hours. Most of this quick access food energy comes from carbohydrates such as fruits, vegetables, breads, cereals, sugars, milk, and milk products. If not burned right away, excess food is stored in the fat cells.

When we run, walk, throw a ball, or dance, our muscles

demand access to instant energy. Glucose in the body is quickly metabolized to provide the ATP that's required. If we need additional glucose, the body, through a series of processes, converts the energy stored in the fat cells into the necessary glucose.

As opposed to aerobics, anaerobic exercise is brief, from a few seconds up to a minute or two, and intense enough to build muscle mass. Exertion, such as weightlifting, breaks down muscle fibers, which are immediately repaired with protein. Repeated repairs generate increased muscle mass. In other words, the more we use our muscles, the stronger they become.

That brings us to HIIT, high-intensity interval training, a spurt of intense cardio followed by low-intensity exercise or rest, as a way to turn the body into a fat-burning, muscle-making machine. In the late 1930s, German coaches and physicians, working to improve the performance of their nation's Olympic athletes, discovered a novel approach to training that significantly increased the fitness and efficiency of the heart. Athletes running a short distance at high speed, then resting, and repeatedly running and resting in intervals, over time, appreciably strengthened their hearts. Using this high-intensity interval training method, German athlete Rudolph Harbig established world records in the 800- and 400-meter runs.

Many of my female clients desire a sculpted, muscular appearance, so I recommend thirty minutes of HIIT, followed by unwinding movements and meditation. Following a short, high intensity workout, the body continues to burn fat at a high rate, because the cells are still taking in lots of oxygen. In addition, these kinds of workouts stimulate muscle-building hormones. Within a month, a cardio-sculpting approach to HIIT aerobics and weight training can result in flatter abs and a tighter butt.

"Love and be open to the movement you choose to do. When you do, it becomes rewarding and pleasurable. Choose movement that brings a smile to your face."
—*Ashly*

12:

Movement for the Fun of It

Using HIIT, Lauren was getting into the shape she desired, but for her, a workout was just that—work. "Why is getting in shape and staying there so hard?" she groused at the end of a session. "Why can't this be fun?" Many clients enjoy their workouts, because they love movement for movement's sake; but, as they say, variety is the spice of life. I found a way for Lauren to supplement the HIIT training she did with me.

At our next appointment, I asked her, "Are you afraid of heights?"

"Not particularly," Lauren responded, somewhat hesitantly. "How high are we talking?"

"As high as a circus trapeze," I said, flashing a wide grin. Locating a trapeze school in the area, I told Lauren about its founder and chief instructor. "Trained as a gymnast, Art mastered the skills of the flying trapeze in Romania, and now has a school not thirty minutes from here. You game?"

Under Art's watchful tutelage, Lauren learned the basics of aerial movement, progressed to more difficult skills, and now "works out" twice a month flying on the trapeze. Movement that's fun is the best kind. I know of several women who have weekend pickup games of Frisbee. Based on the rules of rugby-style football, the women toss the plastic saucers rather than kicking or running with a ball.

A number of Hollywood actresses stay in shape by combining dance moves and acrobatics centered on a stainless steel pole. Pole dancing is quickly becoming a favored fitness form the world over. Climbs and spins, combined with body inversions and lifts, afford a rigorous upper body and core strength workout.

Other women are serious about Hula Hooping. A great way to tone the abs, back, arms, and legs, spinning a plastic hoop around the waist and hips requires skill, stamina, and enthusiasm. Weighted hoops are easier to hula than the kid's toy variety.

In many communities located near rivers or large lakes, sculling clubs are bubbling up. Rowing strengthens the glutes, abs, shoulders, and biceps, and gliding across a still body of water in an early-morning mist can be Zen-terrific.

Beach or sand volleyball, an Olympic sport since the 1990s and an archetype of casual California seaside culture, is now found in most major cities. Some municipal parks have added sand volleyball courts in recent years. Get some friends together, form a couple of teams, and eat sand.

Seek out hiking and rock climbing organizations in your community. It's a fabulous cardio workout, and you can't beat the scenery. For advanced training and muscle-building benefits, hike or climb while wearing a weighted backpack and carrying a pair of stabilizer poles.

Winter does not necessarily preclude outdoor opportunities for fitness. Cross-country skiing and ice skating can help you cut quite a figure. At any time of the year, roller skating is a healthy diversion, providing a cardio workout while toning the lower body.

For Lauren, the trapeze artist, and many others, men and women, fun movement becomes a self-fulfilling prophecy. They get in shape then stay in shape, to do what they love to do, which turns out to be movement opportunities they would never have considered in the first place.

Nontraditional workouts prove the point that movement can be fun. Here are more suggestions: softball, ballet, biking, bowling, canoeing, golf, hockey, unicycling, juggling, roller blading, soccer, swimming, belly dancing, paddle surfing, and using the trampoline. Whatever form of exercise you favor and regardless of how busy you get, stay in a "no excuses" frame of mind by always honoring your appointment with movement. After all, getting in shape and staying fit is about commitment more than your choice of activities or the equipment you acquire.

Equipment can be as simple and inexpensive as a foam roller, fitness ball, and an assortment of tubing or bands. To avoid soreness and release tension, there's nothing better than a foam roller. Priced around thirty-five to fifty dollars, the foam roller is the ticket to develop flexibility and improve performance while reducing injuries. Moving on a foam roller irons out the body's soft tissues, warming you up for subsequent stretching and exercising the major muscle groups. Select a foam roller that's dense enough to support body parts without bruising. You can choose from a number of foam roller techniques. Position the part of your body you want to "work" on top of the foam roller. Use hands and feet to control the amount of body weight pressure placed on the roller. If you feel pain, stop rolling and take a break for about thirty seconds.

I suggest receiving professional instruction before using a foam roller and always consult your physician first. Individuals with heart or vascular diseases or chronic pain are advised not to use a foam roller. Initially, limit the use of the foam roller to about fifteen minutes, consume lots of water before exercising on the foam roller, and use it every other day. Some therapists prescribe foam roller routines to help address back, hip, or knee issues, particularly among those recovering from injuries. Here are some general foam roller instructions:

- Place the foam roller under the soft tissue of the body part you want to stretch or loosen.
- Using the weight of your body, gently roll back and forth across the muscle area to be addressed.
- Take it gradually, and start from the center of your body, working towards arms and legs.
- Pay particular attention to muscles that feel tight.
- Roll over each muscle or body part three or four times until you feel it relax.
- Avoid rolling over bones and joints. Instead, concentrate on the soft tissue.

With instruction and through experimentation and practice, you will be pleased with the results of your foam roller sessions.

Originally adapted by orthopedic doctors in Switzerland as a physical therapy aid, exercise balls came to the United States in the 1980s. Once introduced to the fitness industry, the large plastic balls became a mainstay in health centers, and later, in the home. These inexpensive balls, available in a variety of sizes depending on the user's height, are the basis for dozens of core muscle exercises. Engage a professional trainer to avoid injury and consult a physician before using.

In general, make sure the ball you are using is the proper size for your height, that it is correctly inflated, and allow plenty of floor space free of tables, chairs, or other encumbrances that can cause injury if you lose your balance. If you feel pain while using the ball, stop and take a break.

Lightweight, versatile, and effective, tubes or bands are an affordable alternative to dumbbells and mechanical weight machines, and they store away in a drawer. Take them with you on vacation or when on a business trip. The price is right too, often less than a hundred dollars for a set.

Before using tubes or bands, seek instruction from a professional trainer and consult your physician. Never use tubes or bands that have visible tears or are damaged. Serious injury may result. Keep in mind that the amount of resistance increases the more the tube or band is stretched, and a particular resistance level will not remain stable.

Workout routines using tubes and bands target the major muscle groups such as the abs, back, chest, legs, shoulders, and arms. Adding a door anchor expands your repertoire to include back rows, chest presses, trunk rotations, twisting crunches, pull downs, push downs, and cardiovascular running movements. Anchors can be positioned either at the top of a door or at the bottom, depending on the exercise you desire.

Tubes and bands are color-coded, coming in a number of lengths and resistance strengths. One color may be equivalent to using a five-pound dumbbell, while another color indicates a higher level of resistance similar to a twenty-pound weight.

The decision to use a tube or a band is one of preference. The more durable resistance tubes are manufactured from stretchable plastic or rubber tubing and usually include handles at both ends. Resistance bands are cut from flat sheets of plastic or rubber and also come with attached handles.

You are doing your body well by nourishing it with movement, and medical evidence suggests the best time to exercise is in the afternoon and early evening hours when the body is most flexible and the heart and lungs are at peak performance.

There's a time to eat, a time to sleep, and a time to work the body thanks to our amazing internal, biological clock. Awake at the same time every morning, on the dot, without an alarm clock? Instinctively know when it's time to break for a meal or turn out the lights to sleep? Humans and nearly every mammal on the planet, insects as well, such as the monarch butterfly, are guided through the day by biological clocks that drive the circadian rhythms of our lives. Amazingly, our physical aptitudes, mental wellbeing, and behaviors are on twenty-four- hour cycles that are internally reset every day as the earth turns on its axis. Deep inside the brain, near the optic nerve, is a tiny mass of neurons called the suprachiasmatic nucleus (SCN), the body's master clock, which regulates when we wake up and go to sleep, along with synchronizing hundreds of bodily functions, including the release of hormones and fluctuations in body temperature. For example, by the time evening comes, the SCN has told the brain to secrete melatonin, the hormone that makes us feel tired and sleepy. At the same time, the liver is told to slow the production of sugar since a body at rest does not require high levels of energy.

That brings us back to the best time of the day to exercise. According to Paul Mellick of the Department of Health and Human Performance at the University of St. Thomas, high-intensity exercise is most beneficial later in the day, because muscles and joints are warmed up and blood is flowing. Specifically, the ideal time is between 3 p.m. and 6 p.m., says Michael Smolensky, adjunct professor of biomedical engineering at the University of Texas at Austin. That's when muscle strength is at its highest, joints are most flexible, and lungs are at peak efficiency. It's not a coincidence that most world records in track-and-field athletics and cycling are established in the afternoon and evening hours.

While it is true that medical evidence indicates that exercise is most conducive in the afternoon and evening, many individuals are devoted to the sunrise run on the beach or a before-hitting-the-office workout at the gym. They say movement in the early hours revs them up and gets them going, more than a cup of coffee ever could. When questioned on the subject of exercise time, I urge clients to determine the hour that best meets their schedules and stick with it. We are creatures of habit, so if you always work out at a specific time each day, whether it's in the morning, afternoon, or early evening, keep the routine that is best for you. More important than when you exercise is that you get out there and move.

"Respect the amount of sleep your body requires. Give your body the rest it needs, and it will reply in kind by giving you plenty of energy to fulfill your dreams."
—Ashly

13:

Slumber is Never Time Wasted

We all do it. We all need it. Sleep is essential to our survival as much as breathing and eating, but why do we slumber a number of hours in every twenty-four-hour cycle? It's a mystery that has scientists stumped. According to Harvard Medical School's Division of Sleep Medicine, a number of promising theories have been advanced, but why we need sleep remains unclear. Three primary theories address the issue of sleep, and the answer may be a combination of all three.

Energy Conservation Theory

Research studies confirm our bodily functions significantly slow during hours of sleep. The body temperature drops, we use less energy, and metabolism decreases as much as ten percent. This conservation of energy served our caveman ancestors well. In the darkness of night, it was difficult, if not overly dangerous, to be out hunting for food, so the body adapted the regimen of sleep, a period of inactivity designed to extend scarce food resources.

Restorative Theory

The long-held belief that our bodies repair and rejuvenate during sleep has gained empirical scientific support in recent years. Through animal research studies, we have observed that animals deprived of sleep lose the immune function and die within a few weeks. In both human and animal research, it's a proven fact that during sleep our bodies amass muscle, repair cellular tissue, release growth hormones, and undergo protein synthesis. Our brains use sleep periods to rejuvenate cognitive functioning. For example, during wakefulness, brain activity results in a buildup of adenosine, a chemical byproduct of neuron cellular activity. Once the brain is flooded with adenosine, we feel the urge to sleep, and during sleep, a period of slower neuron activity, we clear the brain of the chemical. As a result, we awake refreshed and alert.

Brain Plasticity Theory

A recent and intriguing theory, brain plasticity relates to a little-understood phenomenon related to the way the structure and organization of the brain undergoes changes. Infants, for instance, sleep about fourteen hours a day, and, as adults, we tend to sleep seven to eight hours. Does sleep help us learn and retain information? Some scientists are convinced our ability to absorb information and memories and later recall them is a function of the brain's "consolidation" facility, the strengthening of neuron connections taking place during sleep.

The theories of sleep help us understand the importance of getting a good night of slumber. In our overworked culture, it's enticing to skip a meal or go without sleep to free up time to accomplish more, but in the long run, denying food and sleep nourishment is a time-waster rather than a time-saver. In the short term, staying up late to complete tasks makes us sluggish, fatigued, dulls the senses, hampers learning, and can make us moody. Chronic sleep deprivation has been shown to lead to obesity, type 3 diabetes, cardiovascular disease, and a shorter life span.

Sleeping less than six hours a night significantly contributes to weight gain, a number of studies have revealed. Among other bodily disruptions, lack of sleep upsets the processing of glucose, the sugar our cells burn for energy. Instead of using the glucose, the body stores the sugars in the fat cells, resulting in weight gain and eventually, obesity. In a kind of vicious circle, sleep deprived, tired individuals reach for sugary snacks for a quick energy boost. The sugar is stored as fat and the person, too fatigued to exercise, craves even more sugary treats.

Other evidence points to a link between sleep disorders and mental distress. Depression and anxiety have been observed in sleep-deprived people, as well as increased stress, feelings of sadness, pessimism, difficulties with relationships, and eruptions of anger.

Fretting about not accomplishing everything that needs to be done, and worries about money, children, a spouse, or any number of matters can result in sleepless nights of tossing and turning. To help "turn off the mind" and get to sleep, nourish your body with regular exercise. A group of insomnia patients were instructed to moderately exercise as part of their daily routines. In a short time, they reported longer and better shuteye at night. In another study, researchers determined moderate activity about six hours before bedtime reduced anxiety and brought on improved sleep.

Avoid eating three hours before hitting the sack. The body needs time to digest the meal before it can rest and repair. Going to sleep on a full stomach can aggravate acid reflux and irritable bowel syndrome. Instead of seeking comfort in food, prepare your body for sleep by turning down the lights, turning off the television, especially the reports of murder and mayhem typical of most late-night news broadcasts, take a warm bath, and listen to soothing music.

Make your "to-do" list for the next day. Getting that information out of your head can help settle the brain for a long-evening nap.

Darken the bedroom. Place the digital clock in a position so the illuminated numerals do not keep you awake. In bed, take several deep breaths, clear the mind of rampaging thoughts, and calm yourself for sleep.

Sometimes we can't stop analyzing events that happened

earlier in our day. The memories of an angry boss, a pushy customer, or a back-stabbing co-worker keep us awake. Replace these memories with pleasant ones, suggests Dr. Charles Pollack, director of the Center for Sleep Medicine at Cornell University's Weill Medical College. Recall a favorite vacation spot, such as a trip to a tropical beach resort. Remember the feel of the warm sand, the refreshing surf, and the visual masterpiece of an evening sunset. Distract your mind with pleasurable thoughts, and sleep will come soon enough, he says.

Nourish your body with the sleep it needs and desires. For most of us, that's seven to nine hours of slumber.

"If the focus of your life is on your purpose, your reason for being here, you tend to eat and move accordingly. When eating and movement principles are aligned with your soul, you can accomplish the things you intend to do."
—Ashly

14:

Nourish the Soul to be Whole

We take time to nourish our bodies by eating healthy, wholesome foods, and we schedule at least an hour a day to nourish our bodies through movement to keep it strong and limber. We give ourselves the sleep we need to restore and renew. As much as the body needs food and thrives on movement and sleep, we also require self-contemplation and meditation to be whole. I know how valuable it has been for my progress to have moments of quiet solitude, a time to be with God to nourish my soul.

Ironically, I was a teenager on the hectic, bustling streets of Shanghai, China when I initially learned the importance of slowing down and enjoying life more fully. A few weeks after high school graduation, I joined a group of American teenagers as a People to People Student Ambassador. Influenced by personally witnessing the destruction of global war, President Dwight Eisenhower started the program as a way to forge bonds of friendship among nations, and, since 1962, college and high school students have toured in Europe, Asia, and other locations, often staying in private homes. I was eighteen when I flew to Oahu for orientation classes at the University of Hawaii. Four days later, our group of young ambassadors landed in Seoul, South Korea. After arriving in the country, I stayed in the rural home of the

Korean National Women's Volleyball Team's coach and his wife. From there, with my group I traveled to Taiwan and Japan, staying in homes and learning the customs of our host families.

Following a stopover in Hong Kong, we entered communist China, flying to Shanghai. Not permitted to stay with a host family, we were housed in a hotel. I experienced a lively city, teeming with millions of people, where the pace was surprisingly slow and low key, especially in the Old Town neighborhoods with men playing cards and mahjong and street vendors cleaning fish and cooking duck.

Here, in this massive metropolis, the people embraced a simpler way of life, and they seemed to slow down to enjoy life's little pleasures. I came to realize that slowing down to become mindful is a choice. We can choose to appreciate the world around us, the tastes, scents, and sights of the everyday, or we can be in such a hurry, focused on the next task, that we miss them all, and, in so doing, never truly experience life's many joys.

Culturally, the religions of the Far East suggest we focus our energies on the most important undertaking, while leaving tasks of less importance to another day, or simply letting them go. By doing less, paradoxically, we do more. Some individuals, especially women, pride themselves on their ability to make lists, often page-after-page inventories of jobs that they feel they need to accomplish. Excessive "to-do list making" usually results in frustration, because there are never enough hours in a day to do it all. Apply "the less is more" philosophy, and you'll be much happier, more content, and satisfied with your achievements. Live in the moment and stop fretting about tomorrow. When we are mindful in the moment, we tend to purchase less, eat less, and worry less.

You will find that with this practice, everything becomes more deliberate, purposeful, and intentional. We eat slowly, and, in so doing, enjoy our food more. We pause to smell the flowers, and, in so doing, contemplate the wonder of a honeybee at work. We take a leisurely walk, and, in so doing, find more pleasure in the natural world. Do less. Live more.

In harmony with nature, we are in the frame of mind to meditate, a way to calm fretfulness and find inner peace. Practiced by Eastern cultures for thousands of years, meditation soothes the mind and relaxes the body. Through meditation, we turn our thoughts away from concerns and worries, replacing anxiety with tranquility. Scientists continue to debate the significance of meditation for our bodies and health, but I am convinced the benefits are legion: stress reduction, self-awareness, and a more positive outlook, all emotional benefits that lead to lower blood pressure, less anxiety, more energy, and deeper, more restful sleep.

We can meditate by visualizing a tranquil scene such as a lake or a snowcapped mountain; by focusing on our breathing and being mindfully aware of our inner consciousness; or by repeating a mantra, a word or a phrase meant to calm the mind. We can be in meditation while sitting quietly, listening to music, seeking communion with God in prayer, or reading and reflecting on the experience itself. Like any skill that's worthwhile, meditation takes practice. Start your meditation exercise gradually, maybe with only a couple of minutes of quiet contemplation. If your mind wanders, and I assure you, it will, gently return the focus to your breathing. Feel your breath. Inhale. Exhale. For most of us, our minds are not accustomed to long stretches of quiet and inactivity, so we must train the mind to enjoy the pleasures of meditation. Give yourself permission to meditate, and your time in self-thought will naturally progress.

I recommend my clients consider Tai chi, qigong, and yoga, three meditation and relaxation disciplines based on traditional Chinese medicine or martial arts.

Combining graceful, purposeful movement with deep breathing, tai chi (pronounced TIE-chee) causes a sense of mental serenity and clarity of thought. Sometimes referred to as "meditation in motion," tai chi involves a series of postures that flow from one to the next. When practiced regularly, tai chi is praised for its ability to diminish stress, increase aerobic capacity, improve balance and agility, tone the muscles, and boost stamina.

Qigong (pronounced chee-gung) is the practice of finding alignment with one's "life energy" through posture, meditative breathing, and mental focus. Some researchers credit qigong with healing certain diseases, lowering blood pressure, reducing anxiety, and enhancing overall quality of life.

A way to rid the mind of "to-do list" anxiety, yoga helps our bodies become more flexible and our minds more composed. Through controlled breathing, a series of stretching moves, and relaxation techniques, yoga is credited with lowering blood pressure and improving heart capacity. A number of yoga poses are quite difficult and require professional training, but several basic poses are safe for the beginner, such as the "mountain pose," "downward dog," and "warrior."

Practicing yoga for a number of years and taking part in my fitness "boot camps," Kayla, a divorced mother of a twelve-year-old daughter, continued to be troubled about her failed marriage. After one of our sessions, she confided, "Ashly, there are times I can't catch a breath. I'm gasping, and I know I'm going to die. I'm so afraid."

"Why are you afraid?" I gently probed.

"I don't know," she stated, tears welling in her eyes. "That's just it. I'm just afraid. My doctor put me on Zoloft for the panic attacks and anxiety, but I don't think that's helping much. I have no one to blame but myself. Tom left me, and I deserved it. I couldn't make him happy, and now I feel my life is spinning out of control."

When I read that Christian author and lecturer Joyce Meyer was scheduled to speak in our area, I ordered a pair of tickets, one for me and the other for Kayla. Meyer's best-selling book, *Battlefield of the Mind*, addresses issues of depression, anger, and anxiety, particularly involving women. According to Meyer, the way we think is how we act. Since our minds are essentially "a battlefield," we are constantly at war, as negative, harmful thoughts fight against positive, life-affirming ones. During the lecture, Meyer, in her down-home style, told her audience that happiness is not a feeling. It is a choice. To be happy, we must choose to be happy rather than respond to the circumstances that tend to control our happiness. Another point in the lecture resonated with Kayla: Meyer's observation that for many people, eighty percent of the problem revolves around how they feel about themselves.

My friend and client, Kayla, is not alone in her self-deprecating approach to life. Many individuals, especially women, spend an inordinate amount of time tearing themselves down rather than building themselves up. In their eyes, they can do nothing right and everything that turns sour is their fault. Joyce Meyer's observation that we can be our own worst critic, especially when we choose to wallow in discontent, is exactly right. Stinkin' thinkin' poisons the mind, hampers the psyche, and often manifests in stress-related illnesses and conditions, including heart disease, diabetes, obesity, gastrointestinal issues, and headaches.

We can change the way we eat, our manner of exercise, and our mind's outlook on life. Neurologists and neurophysicists are only beginning to unlock the science of thought and the untapped potential of the human brain. The acclaimed pathologist Dr. Caroline Leaf and others tell us that what we think directly impacts our health, sense of self, and relationships. Our thought life determines our fortunes and circumstances, and our thoughts take place in an incredible mix of living chemicals and electrical currents acting and reacting at a faster-than-light rate of four-hundred billion a second.

Aerobic exercise changes the heart and lungs by increasing their capacities. Weight training transforms the body's major muscles, making them stronger. Thinking and reasoning stimulates and changes the structure of the brain, expanding its ability to process information, learn, master, remember, and invent. In short, the more you use your gray matter, the greater will be your potential. It stands to reason that positive, life-affirming, optimistic thinking begets more of the same.

"Mental training is what divides the great from the exceptional."
—Ashly

15:

Think Lovely Thoughts

In the Broadway musical adaptation of the timeless J.M. Barrie's *Peter Pan*, we are told to "think lovely thoughts," with the promise that you can soar to places never before seen. Every minute, awake or asleep, our minds click along, popping out thoughts by the thousands, so we need to ask ourselves:

"Do the thoughts I have benefit me?"

"Do they support my goals?"

"Do they enhance my relationships?"

"Do they make me a better, more understanding, and compassionate person?"

"Do they nourish me with spiritual food?"

The thoughts we think, are they lovely? Consider this often-voiced thought: "I need to lose weight, so I can fit in this outfit." There's nothing lovely about clothes that are too tight, and thinking like this is downright ugly. It's demeaning and degrading. This thought certainly fails to promote wellness. Admonishing oneself for being too fat or not thin enough is counterproductive. This is "stinkin' thinkin'" that makes you feel less worthy.

A praiseworthy thought would be: "I nourish myself through the foods I eat, the movement my body desires, and the time I give myself." Rather than issuing a "put down," give yourself a "lift up." Turn the negative into the positive, pessimism into optimism, hopelessness into hopefulness, and a frown into a smile.

As part of my group fitness and body transformation classes, we work on improving our mental strength, our mind's capability to meet life's challenges head-on and overcome obstacles. In the heat of an aerobics workout, we enthusiastically call out inspiring, positive words, and as these words, coming from many voices, reverberate about the room, energy and a feeling of power lifts the spirits of all. What are these words? Here are some I often hear:

"I'm strong!"

"I'm sexy!"

"I'm more than capable!"

"I'm amazing!"

These women, determined to concentrate on their ideal selves, are retraining their minds to think lovely thoughts. They are building mental strength. A credit to the power of a strong-willed mind, when we think positive, uplifting thoughts, we can do more. I have seen this time and again. Clients easily increase repetitions or lift more weight when they believe they can. Saying, "I can't," weakens the body. Believing "I can," empowers the muscles.

My client, Arianna, described it this way: "I'm working my abs, I'm burning, and they hurt so badly. I don't think I can go another rep, but then I bring mindfulness into play, focus on being strong, visualizing the abs and my entire body becoming one. I find an inner strength to do more reps and I'm tougher for it."

Coaches and sports psychologists often talk about mental toughness, the willfulness that comes from deep inside the mind that makes us press on, persevere, perform at our very best, and never give up. Some athletes claim you are born with mental toughness, but in my experience, it is a learned trait that makes us determined, focused, and confident. In the extreme, mental toughness is Diana Nyad pushing herself to complete a 110-mile open-ocean swim from Cuba to Florida, or Michael Jordan, stricken with the flu and near total collapse from exhaustion, making the winning shot in the 1997 NBA finals.

Most of us will not attempt a long-distance swim or compete at the level of NBA professionals, but training our minds to be mentally tough will make us more resilient in the gym, on the job, and in the home. Mental toughness begins with goal setting, determining what you want to accomplish and why. Goals need to be doable as well as challenging, so raise the figurative bar, but not beyond the possibility of human endurance. Specific, measurable goals are better than ones that are vague or general in nature.

Following the birth of her first child, Arianna came to me to help her flatten her belly. "I'm close to getting back to my pre-birth weight," she told me, "but my abs leave a lot to be desired. You see, I'm a swimsuit model and I want to get back to work."

"Do you have a photo of yourself showing your abs before your pregnancy?"

Arianna smiled. "I do. I'll bring it to our next session."

The following week, Arianna, as promised, brought a magazine cover of herself posing in a yellow bikini on a beach, and indeed, her abs were picture-perfect. Since she had a workout space in her home, I suggested she post the magazine cover at eye-level. "Under the cover, position this index card," I continued, giving her a blank card and a marker. "Let's take a moment to write down your goal and why it's important to you, because a big part of goal-setting success is determining your reasons, your 'why.'"

Arianna wrote: "My goal is to have abs like this. Why? I want to work again doing what I love."

Prescribing a workout routine of dumbbell pushups, squats, curls, lunges, and similar exercises, I helped Arianna put together a day-to-day and week-to-week schedule of increasing repetitions.

"When the going gets tough," I advised, "recall your goal, your 'why,' by looking at the magazine cover, and follow up with lots of positive self-talk." Like when giving yourself a pep talk, thoughts of affirmation channel our thinking, encourage us to persist, and muster the will to go on. Here are examples of Arianna's self-talk:

"I am growing stronger by the minute."

"I am building picture-perfect abs with every rep."

"I am confident and beautiful."

"I believe in me."

Through self-talk, we train our brains to believe what we wish and our bodies follow. Repeat these and similar statements in your self-talk affirmations:

"I am focused on my goals."

"I am determined to succeed."

"I am strong and capable."

"I am at my best."

We can borrow a technique favored by many of the world's preeminent athletes. Visualization, seeing in your mind what you expect to accomplish, sharpens mental acuity and heightens confidence. "Scripting" their visualizations, elite athletes write in detail the thoughts and actions required to win a sprint on the cinder track or race in the snow against the clock on a downhill course. An estimated eighty percent of Olympic track and field athletes practice visualization before and during meets. Two-time Olympic medalist and three-time world record holder in the men's high jump, Dwight Stones, seconds before an event, visibly stepped through the mechanics of the leap, later explaining he was tossing out distractions to focus on visualizing his imminent performance. Mental rehearsals teach the mind to concentrate and focus like a champion.

One of the world's loveliest men is a Buddhist monk, born and educated in Central Vietnam in the years before the American involvement in that nation's conflicts. Thich Nhat Hahn (pronounced tic not han) often writes and speaks on the subject of finding harmony and happiness through practiced mindfulness. From his residence in a monastery situated in the South of France, this gentle monk has published more than one hundred books and travels the world as a lecturer and activist for peaceful solutions to international conflicts. He studied comparative religions at Princeton University, was a lecturer at Columbia University, and established a number of Buddhist monasteries throughout the world, including several in the United States. His book, *Living Buddha, Living Christ*, was a 1995 best seller.

Nhat Hanh defines mindfulness as the energy of life, an awareness of your environment, being present and at one with those around you, and in touch with what you are doing. Mindfulness is a source of happiness, he says, when we touch life deeply in every moment of our lives. Tasks as mundane as shopping for groceries, preparing meals, and washing dishes, when performed mindfully, become joyful, because we are living in the here and now, our senses alert, and curiosity wide awake.

When practicing mindful eating, drinking, and consuming, Nhat Hanh says we nourish our minds and bodies in four ways, namely through the foods we eat; our ability to see, taste, and feel the world around us; how we choose to act, interact and react; and our conscious awareness. Interviewed by Oprah Winfrey for her magazine, Nhat Hanh said, "Many people are alive, but don't touch the miracle of being alive."

Most people, Oprah observed, busy going from one thing to the next, often overwhelmed with everyday chores, seldom take time to realize the precious gift of life.

"That is the environment people live in," Nhat Hanh responded. "But with practice, we can always remain alive in the present moment. With mindfulness, you can establish yourself in the present in order to touch the wonders of life that are available in that moment. It is possible to live happily in the here and now. So many conditions of happiness are available—more than enough for you to be happy right now. You don't have to run into the future in order to get more."

Oprah requested an example of experiencing happiness in the moment.

"Suppose you are drinking a cup of tea," clarified Nhat Hanh. "When you hold your cup, you may like to breathe in, to bring your mind back to your body, and you become fully present. And when you are truly there, something else is also there—life, represented by the cup of tea. In that moment, you are real, and the cup of tea is real. You are not lost in the past, in the future, in your projects, in your worries. You are free from all of these afflictions. In that state of being free, you enjoy your tea. That is the moment of happiness and of peace. When you brush your teeth, you may have just two minutes, but, according to this practice, it is possible to produce freedom and joy during that time, because you are established in the here and now. If you are capable of brushing your teeth in mindfulness, then you will be able to enjoy the time when you take a shower, cook your breakfast, sip your tea."

Nhat Hanh urges us to train our minds to appreciate the present. Once mindful of our thoughts, we live a lovelier life.

"Thoughts lead to feelings which lead to behaviors. Before a thought takes root, we have a choice to believe it or not."
—*Ashly*

16:

What is True? What is Not?

"I'll never get the weight off," Chelsea lamented. "I'm going to be fat and overweight for the rest of my life. I guess I was made this way, and that's the way it is."

A newer member of one of my fitness classes, Chelsea was venting to another of my clients, Britta. Overhearing the outburst, I asked Chelsea to stay a moment after class.

"I couldn't help seeing that you're hurting, Chelsea," I opened the conversation. "Tell me why you're discouraged."

"I've been on so many different diets and exercise programs that I lost count long ago," she sobbed. "I get rid of some of the weight, but it always comes back, and when it does, I'm heavier than before. I'm a lost cause. I may as well give up. I don't even know why I signed up for your class."

When I motioned to a chair, Chelsea sat down, and I pulled up a chair beside her. "Let's slow down," I suggested. "Take a deep breath." She did. "Let's take another. Breathe it in and then let it out, nice and slow." Chelsea followed my lead.

"You'll never get the weight off," I stated. "Does that statement resonate with you to be true?"

"Of course, it's true," she practically screamed. "I know my body," she moaned. Taking in another breath to calm herself, she quietly affirmed what she told Britta. "I will never get the weight off. There, I said it. I'm going now."

She started to get up, and again I motioned for her to remain seated. "Let's sit and breathe with that thought for a moment or two more," I said. "You'll never get the weight off. Does that statement resonate with you to be true?"

"I'm afraid it does. I've always been heavy and always will be. It's the way I was made."

"Let's sit with this thought a bit more, breathe, and take a second look at it."

Noticeably agitated, Chelsea muttered, "I don't see the purpose of this." Again she said, "I will never get the weight off. That's what's true."

"Has there been a time in your life when you were thinner than you are now?"

"Yes, I've had some success."

I asked, "You'll never get the weight off. Is that unquestionably true?"

"I guess not," she sighed.

I pressed on. "Let's sit with this for a moment more, Chelsea. Let me ask you, 'How would you visualize yourself, if you knew you could have the body you want?'"

"That's easy," she smiled. "I'd feel okay with myself."

It was my turn to smile. "Let's sit and breathe in those thoughts, those good feelings." Then, I asked Chelsea to come up with a positive thought, an affirmation, about her feelings at that very moment.

"I feel better about myself. I feel empowered."

My smile broadened and I nodded.

"I get it," Chelsea said. "I can feel good about myself at this moment, and I have the power to change, if I want to change."

"That's right."

"And when I feel good about myself, I'm no longer defeated."

Our smiles turned to laughter. As Chelsea departed the fitness room, I detected a lift in her step that I think reflected her heart.

Getting to the heart of the matter, clearing the mind of unrelated clutter, and zeroing in on positive thinking is a potent technique introduced by Byron Katie, a suicidal, self-loathing, twice-divorced mother of three who had her eureka moment in a rundown Los Angeles halfway house for women with eating disorders. Growing up in and around Barstow, California, Byron Kathleen Reid preferred to be called Katie. She attended Northern Arizona University for a few months but dropped out to marry her boyfriend. After three children and a divorce, Katie remarried and, again living in Barstow, was a depressed mess, eating too much, hating herself, and considering suicide her only way out.

She checked herself in to the L.A. halfway house, but the other women refused to room with her. Katie's fiery temper and irate rants terrified the residents, who relegated her to a bed set up in the attic. Believing she was unworthy of a mattress, she curled up on the attic floor, painfully alone, confused, and angry. Awakened by a cockroach crawling over her foot, this pitiful woman says she saw herself as others would have seen her at that moment. According to Katie, that morning she gave herself permission to end the nightmare that had become her existence. What was the turnaround? She realized that when she believed the worst about herself, she was in pain, but when she objectively questioned her perceived shortcomings, she no longer suffered. In fact, by changing her thinking, she transformed her life. Through her writings, workshops, school, and public speaking, "The Work of Byron Katie" has touched the lives of millions.

Inspired by Bryon Katie's "The Work," I have helped clients, such as Chelsea, gain clarity. Self-loathing is no way to live. It certainly does not lead to healing. Introspective questioning that challenges our opinions of ourselves often does. Here are the questions:

Does it resonate true?

Is it unquestionably true?

How do you feel when you believe it is true?

How would you visualize yourself, if that idea had never entered your mind?

What affirmation comes to mind at this moment?

These five questions, combined with purposeful breathing, visualization, mindfulness, and self-talk, change attitudes, alter perceptions, and turn negative and toxic beliefs into positive, self-affirming actions. Hopeful people embrace life and nourish the body and soul.

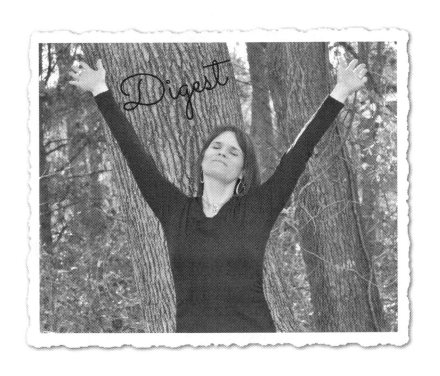

Digest

PART 3

"The way we digest our thoughts, experiences, and beliefs is the way we digest our foods."
—Ashly

17:

My Search for Balance

In the **END Zone**, we learn to embrace and nourish ourselves. We want to live our best lives, experience happiness and pleasure in everything, and fulfill our purpose, but these affirmations can come about only when the body and mind are in balance. Since the way we digest our thoughts, experiences, and beliefs is the way we digest our foods, the ideal state of digestion is one of physical and emotional harmony. Only when our body is in a relaxed state can complete digestion and assimilation occur, because the stress response automatically hinders the digestive system or shuts it down.

At one time or another, we've all experienced the tightening of the stomach muscles when we are upset, angry, or frightened. In the extreme, the stomach may empty its contents, preparing the body to either fight or run, reactions dating back to our early ancestors' drive to survive in a hostile world. We no longer battle fearsome saber-tooth tigers, but we still have fears and worries, and these anxieties manifest themselves in the way we digest our foods.

We go through our day hungry for acceptance, approval, compassion, kindness, and love—a warm embrace, a thoughtful word, a smile of recognition. It's as instinctive as a young child's hug and as essential to our happiness as the food we eat, water we consume, and air we breathe. It took years for me to slow down and fully listen to my body, let go of debilitating angst, and value myself for who I am.

A freshman at Abilene Christian University, I was a fashion merchandising major and, as much as I loved clothes and dreamed of working in New York's fashion district, I was all thumbs in the sewing room. Accidentally slicing a hole through the shirt I was making, I hurriedly patched it with tape to avoid failing the class project. The business school curriculum was no better. If balance sheets, income statements, accounts payables and receivables did not leave me spinning, the basics of economics, elasticity, price systems, and supply and demand certainly did.

A daily requirement at ACU, chapel was a thirty-minute time of praise and worship. All campus classes and activities came to a halt so the student body could gather at Moody Coliseum. Habitually late, I found a seat near the center aisle, two or three rows from the front. There was this good-looking, first-year football player, Robert Torian, I'd seen in one of my classes, but we had not spoken. Apparently, he noticed me, too, and, as I later learned, looked for me each day at chapel.

Another ACU tradition, this one dating to 1918, was Lectureship, an annual three-day event involving thousands of participants who gathered for lectures and workshops covering biblical and religious themes. To my surprise and joy, Robert asked me to accompany him to our freshman year Lectureship. At the end of the first day's program, we went to dinner and started dating. Of course, we shared our thoughts about classes, and what he was doing in his major field of study, Adult Corporate Fitness, sure sounded more fun than basic business and trying to make accounting entries balance. Dropping my business major, I joined Robert as a student of Adult Corporate Fitness to learn about organic and biological chemistry, nutrition, physiology, and personal training.

After landing a summer job as an aerobics instructor at an athletic club near my parents' home, I met Terry Doherty, a tall, lanky, athletic woman who turned out to have a heart of gold. A program director at the club, Terry took me under her wing and for two summers, mentored and encouraged me to become a personal trainer. Twelve years my senior, Terry not only instructed me on helping clients become fitter, but also taught me the business side of her work. After graduation and marrying Robert, I joined Terry in the business as one of her company's full time trainers, staying with her for three years. In 1991, Robert and I had our first child, Clinton. At first, I took Clinton to work with me to client appointments, but, as the months went on, working ten-hour days and caring for a baby became too much. Perceptive as always, Terry knew I was struggling to keep up with the demands of motherhood and a full-time job. I preferred not to leave Clinton in daycare, so Terry generously made it possible for me to strike out on my own. Continuing to work with two of my long-term clients, each three days a week, I became a part-time personal trainer and business owner. Twenty months after our first child's birth, Brandon was born. By this time, Robert was employed as a warehouse manager, a job he did not enjoy, but it paid most of the household bills.

I was fortunate to find a wonderful lady who watched the children a few hours a day while I continued my business, and, when Clinton entered first grade, and Brandon was in kindergarten, the personal training business organically grew. Clients told family and friends about me, and soon I had a full-time business that I worked around the children's school schedules. A big-time overachiever, I was constantly on the go, volunteering at Clinton and Brandon's elementary school, serving as an officer of the parent-teacher organization, training clients, being a wife, and taking care of the house. "I can push through anything," was my attitude. "Let me take on more. My body can handle it. I'm invincible."

For a weekend get-together involving my parents, brothers, sisters, their kids and our family, I volunteered to shop for all the food. This was for five families, mind you, but I was convinced I was on top of it. At the supermarket, I pushed two carts, each heaping with provisions. Back home, I cooked and baked, and we loaded the food and our two young children in the car for the one-hour trip to my parents' ranch.

Within minutes upon arriving, I felt a burning pain shoot across my back. It forced me to my knees. Instantly intensifying, the pain, wrapping around my rib cage, squeezed the breath out of me. I was on the ground, panicking in terror, unable to breathe and losing consciousness as my brain silently screamed, "Oh, my goodness, what is happening to me?"

My husband, the burly, former football player, taking me in his arms, lifted me off the ground. I caught a breath, but it wasn't easy, and, if I sat, I still gasped for air. Over the course of the day, the excruciating, fiery pain abated a little and I could breathe easier, but it persisted in my middle back. The next twelve months were a blur of pain and panic. I was functioning as a mom while keeping the business going, but barely. The memories of that year are few: puppet shows with my kids out in the yard and, at the end of the day, Robert holding and comforting me. Good at masking the pain, I kept the turmoil inside, away from the children and my clients, but my husband, mother, and my sister Jamie knew better. The feelings of anxiousness and fear continued for a period of four years.

Gradually, I could no longer exercise my upper body and arms, only my legs. The doctors, baffled by my deterioration, wanted to put me on heavy-duty painkillers, but not one to medicate myself with prescription drugs, I tried yoga and other forms of meditation, and these techniques worked to an extent, but I was still in pain.

Unable to lift any appreciable weight with my arms and upper body, I sought the counsel of one of the best physical therapists in the nation, Dave Bloom. Not long ago, Dave lost his battle with Stage IV Mestatic Melanoma, but when I knew him, he was at the top of his profession. "What's wrong with me?" I pleaded.

His prognosis was a stunner: "Ashly, physically there's nothing at all wrong with you," he stated. "It is a soul issue."

"A soul issue?" I sputtered. "How can I have a soul issue?" I asked, in disbelief. "I don't have issues with God. I went to a Christian university. I took Bible classes. I pray and talk to God all the time. How could I have a soul issue?"

"The soul is the mind, your heart, and emotions," Dave enlightened me. "And they all tie in together to make us who we are. They encase our fears and strengths, anxieties and courage. Everything we think about and how we take in the world around us is assimilated into our being." According to Dave Bloom, fears and anxiety had set up shop inside me and now manifested themselves as physical pain and weakness. Rid myself of the anxiety, and the pain would soon follow, he advised.

Nearly every evening before bedtime, I read to my elementary-aged boys stories from a children's Bible. It was a beautifully illustrated book, a retelling of Jesus' life, such as the story of feeding the five thousand, the miracles of calming the sea and walking on water, and healing the sick little girl. Our favorite story was about the ailing woman who believed if she just could touch the robe of Jesus, she would be healed.

On one particular morning, the routine began the same as it was every school day. Robert left for work. The children and I ate breakfast and walked together the few blocks to their school. I checked to make sure they had their lunches, hugged them each goodbye, and returned to the house. Pulling out of the driveway later in the morning, I expected to make the thirty-minute commute to the Irving, Texas YMCA and the session with my first client of the day.

On the radio, a Michael Jackson song was playing as I steered onto Texas 121, the busy highway that bisects the massive Dallas/

Fort Worth International Airport. Before I hit the mammoth toll plaza, a massive ball of energy swooped out of my gut, electrified my chest, and seemed to want to explode out of me. In a rush of anxiety and emotion, my brain screamed, "Run! Get Away!" With my heart pounding, uncontrollable breaths coming in gulps, throat tightening, the body quaking wildly, I raised my right hand heavenward and cried out in prayer, "Lord, I cannot do this another day. I can't feel this way anymore. Can I touch you? Can you reach down to me? Can we meet in the middle? Please take this away from me, so I don't have to experience it anymore. I'm done. I give you control."

At that instant, I saw Jesus in my mind, his hand extended to my hand, and my body was instantly at peace. The drive through the airport toll booths, the highways to Irving, and the streets to the YMCA left only vague impressions. In my parking spot at the Y, I thought, "Wow, it's gone." After four years of anxiety attacks, that was the last one. That morning, I turned control of my life over to God. There was no more back pain. My arm strength rapidly returned.

Strange thing about irrational fear and anxiety, it can be gone for a very long time, and then begin to reappear, taking a different form. So it was with me. Seven years had passed since that morning on Texas 121 when I was set free. The boys were in middle school, and I was in my forties. Eating an apple at home one evening, I felt my throat thicken and become tight. I convinced myself I had become allergic to apples, and that was a shame, because I loved apple cake, apple pie, apple cobbler, anything made with apples; but nevertheless, I eliminated apples from my diet. Next, I experienced tightness in my throat while eating peanut butter, again a favorite since childhood. Some people are deathly allergic to peanuts, so I convinced myself I was allergic to peanuts too.

In a twenty-four-month period, I imagined allergic reactions to wheat products, rice products, and other foods until I had eliminated entire food groups. Fearing food allergies, I no longer ate in restaurants, and I limited myself to less than fifteen food choices. Conferring with psychologists was not helpful, but I knew I had a problem and needed help. Seeking to know the reason this was happening to me, I researched food issues and became familiar with the Institute for the Psychology of Eating (IPE). Founded in Boulder, Colorado by an expert in nutritional medicine, Marc David, IPE certifies eating psychology coaches in a number of disciplines such as body image, weight issues, compulsive eating, unwanted eating habits, and digestive challenges. Having begun to earn my institute certification, I connected with one of their knowledgeable food coaches, Cynthia Stadd, a Boulder resident and owner of Eat Empowered. At the same time, I sought out Angela Adkins, who practiced the Body Talk System, a holistic therapy that allows your internal energy system to be "resynchronized." Combining Body Talk with food coaching was like healing on steroids, but without the drugs.

Using Body Talk, Angela helped me clear out the trash, the toxic ideas that had promoted fears and anxieties within me, and Cynthia educated me about nutrition and digestion in ways that fundamentally altered my belief system. In short, I was experiencing a powerful one-two punch of healing by taking out the bad and putting in the good. Finding balance in my life, I was about to move into the **END Zone.**

"You've got to take out the trash before you can bring in the good stuff."
—*Ashly*

18:

Some Gut Wisdom to Ponder

My search to understand our body's ability to assimilate not only food and drink, but also the observations and lessons, good and bad, making up who we are is what turned my life around. A big step in my healing resulted from Body Talk, the holistic approach pioneered by Dr. John Veltheim. Trained as a chiropractor and traditional acupuncturist, this former martial arts instructor in Australia is the author of nine books on acupuncture, Reiki, and Body Talk. According to Body Talk proponents, the body's energy networks can be brought into harmony through physical manipulation. Healing occurs when the Body Talk practitioner assists the body's natural processes to come into synchronization through "muscle-bio feedback."

Veltheim's wife, Esther, created Body Talk's "BreakThrough System," a seven-step process of self-inquiry that challenges one's deep-seated beliefs. Each of us harbors entrenched, possibly subconscious, beliefs about ourselves, and these beliefs tend to prevent us from reaching our full potential. The idea is to get these beliefs out in the open, determine if they are harmful or toxic, and if they are unwanted, clear them from our psyche.

Through Body Talk and the "BreakThrough System," I

realized I could not be my true, authentic self until I rid myself of fears and anxieties based on deep-seated, toxic beliefs, many of them dating back to childhood. Meanwhile, Cynthia Stadd coached me through the toxic beliefs I had about food and helped me integrate a new belief system.

According to Cynthia, since physical digestion is a reflection of an individual's ability to digest life, therefore, in order to address issues with food, I needed to confront my fears. In addition to coaching me about diet, Cynthia encouraged me to dig deep into thoughts, beliefs, and emotions that hindered my ability to eat with pleasure, love, and joy. With her help, I became aware of irrational beliefs that manifested as allergies such as to apples or peanuts, and I realized that I tended to internalize fears brought on by feelings of inadequacy and low self-esteem.

I continued my studies at the Institute for the Psychology of Eating, where I learned that the stomach and digestive system are much more than food processors. They also help us digest our thoughts, observations, and emotions.

We hear terms such as "gut wisdom," "gut instinct," and "listen to your gut," and we are all familiar with having a "nervous stomach" or "butterflies," because we have a "gut feeling" about something that could be "gut wrenching." Attaching intelligence to the entrails is not simply a matter of colloquial language. There's real science behind it. Until fairly recently, the belly's enteric nervous system was thought to regulate the digestion and assimilation of foods and beverages, and that's about it. It turns out, this mass of neurons and neurotransmitters functioning as an auxiliary brain in conjunction with the one in our head, plays a big part in determining our emotions.

Research conducted at the Department of Anatomy and Cell Biology at New York-Presbyterian Hospital/Columbia University Medical Center has determined this "second brain," while not capable of solving a math problem or composing a novel, contains as many as one-hundred million neurons, impressive enough to function with its own reflexes and senses independently of the brain in the skull cavity. In fact, some ninety percent of the fibers in the visceral nerve that connects the gut with the brain travel in one direction, meaning the gut sends much more data to the head than the other way around.

What is the subject matter of all this communication? Apparently, gut chemistry has an impact on behavior, emotions, moods, and our responses to stressful information, suggest scientists at Hamilton, Ontario's McMaster University. Taking into account the gut's ability to communicate with the brain, "it's almost unthinkable that the gut is not playing a critical role in mind states," observed Dr. Emeran Mayer, a noted gastroenterologist and director of the Center for Neurobiology of Stress at the University of California, Los Angeles.

Clearly the gut is a barometer of our emotions. When we become upset, angry, or anxious, our gut lets us know in no uncertain terms. It's the feeling of indigestion following a funeral or the gut-wrenching sight of a serious auto accident. These examples are at the extreme end of the soul and digestion spectrum, but they illustrate a truth: We can't separate our emotions and thoughts from our bodily functions, and, in turn, fitness, health, and happiness are dependent on embracing who we are, the nutrition we give ourselves, and how we assimilate the world in which we live into our lives.

The author of several books on nutrition and founder of the Institute for the Psychology of Eating, Marc David suggests that how we eat is as important to our wellbeing as what we eat. Dining without stress, eating slowly and mindfully, enhances digestion and improves metabolism. As a result, we have more energy and are less likely to pack on extra pounds. According to David, issues we have with eating and weight are directly connected to our relationships, family dynamics, career success, concerns about money, sexuality, and issues with intimacy and love, among other matters, and influence our body's physiology, particularly digestion, assimilation, and metabolism. Our thoughts and emotions, feelings of pleasure or sense of unhappiness, the awareness of the foods we eat, and every aspect of our lives determine to a great degree the body's ability to process food efficiently.

In our hurry-up-get-it-done society, rushing to appointments, tossing down food as fast as we can to stay on schedule, dashing to fulfill never-ending obligations, checking off the next line on the endless to-do list, and missing meals, when we finally eat, perhaps late at night, we are voracious, mindlessly shoving in food to stave off hunger pangs. On top of this stress, we heap on the fear, anxiety, self-judgment, and toxic thoughts about ourselves and others that fill our minds on a daily basis.

A body experiencing such relentless stress is not performing at its best. Far from it, stressful lifestyles tax the heart, raise blood pressure, and strain every bodily function, including digestion and assimilation.

What happens when we significantly reduce the stress, breathe, and take life a little slower? In a relaxed state, our body is best able to burn the energy we provide through food, operate at maximum metabolic efficiency, and not have a need to add to the fat stores. Bottom line: Eating under stress makes us heavier; eating while relaxed makes us thinner.

Happy people metabolize their meals more efficiently than their discontented, dissatisfied counterparts, so it stands to reason that if you are on a restrictive, unsatisfying diet, fretting about losing weight, disappointed in your progress, self-loathing and hypercritical of yourself, despite the low-calorie fare, your stressed metabolism is at a disadvantage. Rather than submitting yourself to extreme, bland dietary foods, it's more to your benefit to eat tasty, nutritious foods slowly and mindfully, delighting in every bite, enjoying the aromas, flavors, and textures. The meal is a pleasure, not a responsibility.

Researchers tell us that taking pleasure in eating some foods, for example, flavorful, spicy foods, as well as finding pleasure in a number of other activities, such as making love and orgasm, feeling a sense of excitement, moving the body by playing a sport or exercising, meditating and practicing mindful breathing, and experiencing moments of happiness, all these are linked to the production of endorphins within the pituitary gland.

So what are endorphins, and how do they help us burn the energy stored in fat? As neurotransmitters, endorphins are part of the body's internal communications system, passing signals from one neuron to the next. Some endorphins help us deal with pain, but others help us feel pleasure and give a sense of satisfaction. There is some evidence that when we are the happiest, endorphins signal our body's fat storage to release food that is converted into glucose and burned to make ATP as energy. We may see a toddler walk for the first time. This elation we then feel, triggered by endorphins, results in a burst of ATP energy, and since we are at rest, that energy comes from fat storage. We may admire a stunning work of art. Again, the pleasure results in burning ATP from fat. Every delightful activity, reacting to a funny scene in a movie, holding hands in a park, or anticipating making love when lights are low are all enhanced by endorphins. In turn, endorphins help us burn the energy stored in fat deposits.

Marc David terms this sense of pleasure and its powerful effect on metabolism, "Vitamin P." Humans are wired to seek pleasure and avoid pain, so when we eat, we seek the pleasure of our food while avoiding the pain of being hungry. However, if we hurriedly gulp down the food, even if it's a delicious pizza, at the end of the meal, we see the empty pizza pan and wonder, "Where did it go?" We did not enjoy it, did not taste it, and did not have a pleasurable experience. In fact, we are still hungry, so we order a second pizza. However, if we had mindfully, slowly eaten a slice of pizza, relished the scents of the toppings, taken pleasure in the diversity of flavors and variety of textures, we would have been satisfied. Since the single slice of pizza brought pleasure, it was enough. Here is the takeaway from the pizza shop example: Seek more pleasure from the food you eat, rather than eating more food in a vain attempt to seek pleasure. The slower we eat, the more pleasure we experience during the meal. That's some "gut wisdom" worth pondering.

"Diet companies tell us food is the enemy. That's ridiculous. Food is nourishing, pleasurable, and appears everywhere. It can't be avoided. Instead of hiding from it, be open to a fulfilling relationship with it. Nourish the body and soul through the food you choose to eat, the movement your body desires, and the quiet moments that feed the soul."
—Ashly

19:

Digestion Is Far From a Simple Matter

On the surface, the matter of digestion, taking in food, churning it around, removing nutrients, and getting rid of the waste, appears simple enough. Under the surface, the science is a fascinating tribute to the body's seemingly infinite levels of complexity. A little understanding of digestion basics goes a long way in determining the best foods we need to be eating.

Throughout the day, we expend energy, walking and talking, thinking and working, eating and relaxing. In a typical day, we use about ten percent of our energy quotient digesting and assimilating the foods we eat, but we can increase this percentage based on our diet. For example, proteins require twice the energy to digest than carbohydrates and twenty times more energy than fats. There's ample research that indicates whole foods require more energy to digest than processed foods, another reason to prefer non-processed food products.

The digestive system kicks in the moment foods cross our lips. In the mouth, the teeth grind the food to a pulp, which is mixed with saliva to add moisture, and the tongue kneads the pulp into a ball small enough to be swallowed. Taste buds, thousands of receptors located on the tongue, inform the brain whether the food is sweet or sour, salty or bitter. Infants quickly learn to enjoy pleasurable scents and tastes, and that stimulation of the lips and mouth indicates food is on the way, all of which trigger saliva production. Simply the thought of food becomes a learned response that scientists call the conditioned salivary reflex.

Saliva, composed of water, enzymes, proteins, free amino acids, and inorganic ions similar to the content of blood plasma, chemically interacts with any foods containing starches to begin breaking these foods down into sugar for quick energy.

Swallowing occurs when chewing momentarily halts, breathing slows, and the tongue forces the ball of food into the throat, where powerful muscles contract and squeeze, driving the food through a circular muscle that serves as a kind of flap, into the ten-inch-long esophagus. It takes about ten seconds for the food ball to arrive at the bottom of the esophagus, where another circular muscle relaxes, allows food to pass into the stomach, then closes to inhibit the stomach contents from escaping. However, this tension-sensitive muscle can open to permit the release of gas, as a belch, or stomach contents in the form of vomit.

In the stomach, which can hold about a quart of food and liquids, food is ground into small particles and mixed with gastric juices, and the digestion of carbohydrates and proteins begins. In the gastric juices are various acids; pepsin, the enzyme that helps digest protein; the hormone gastrin, involved in producing energy throughout the body at the cellular level; and serotonin. Blood rushes to the stomach to distribute glucose and other simple sugars, amino acids, and some fats to cellular tissue.

Periodically, a portion of the now semi-liquid mixture is discharged into the small intestine, measuring about twenty-three feet in length with an estimated absorption surface of 5,400 square yards, enough to cover about eighty-five percent of a football field. Here is where carbohydrates, proteins, and fats are further broken down into nutrients such as the calcium, iron, and vitamins essential for healthy living. These chemical reactions requiring digestive enzymes and hormones provided by the pancreas, liver, and gallbladder, act on proteins, carbohydrates, and fats. The liver is a complex gland that produces a number of bodily functions. Regarding digestion, this largest of the glands aids the metabolism of protein, fats, and carbohydrates, which is turned into glucose. This ready supply of energy-rich glucose remains in the liver for about eight to ten hours.

What is left travels as a liquid into the large intestine, a five-foot absorption machine. In the large intestine, most of the liquid is absorbed along with the electrolytes, sodium and chloride. Bacteria synthesize a number of critical nutrients such as niacin and thiamin. Waste materials, carried from the body's cellular tissue, combined with dead bacteria and anything that could not be digested, form feces. Once or twice a day, the waste material is defecated.

It should come as no surprise that the healthiest foods on the planet are the easiest to digest and most beneficial in their natural form. For fitness and health, expand your grocery list with selections from my "Real Foods Meal Planning Guide."

Apples—One a day keeps the doctor away. High in fiber, especially pectin, a soluble fiber that lowers blood cholesterol, the apple is a storehouse of nutrients, including quercetin, an anti-inflammatory. Apples are an outstanding source of disease-fighting antioxidants, compounds that repair oxidation damage at the cellular level. Eat the peel, too, to get ursolic acid, a nutrient that's been shown to combat obesity. Recent studies indicate apples may be useful in preventing Alzheimer's disease.

Artichoke Hearts—High in antioxidants and packed with fiber for digestive health, artichoke hearts lower cholesterol. The potassium helps the heart maintain a healthy rhythm and may reduce the risk of stroke. Phytonutrients boost the immune system.

Avocado—An excellent source of vitamin C, vitamin E, and potassium, avocados aid in the body's absorption of healthy monononsaturated fat, lycopene, and beta-carotene, an antioxidant studied for its ability to thwart prostate cancer, heart disease, and afflictions of the eyes. The carotenoids provide anti-inflammatory benefits.

Bananas—For heart and bone health, normal blood pressure, and muscle function, select bananas for your diet, rich in potassium and high in fiber. In addition, bananas contain a compound that nourishes the beneficial bacteria operating in the digestive system. These bacteria are instrumental in the production of vitamins and digestive enzymes.

Beans—High in heart-healthy fiber, beans are a source of protein as well as iron, potassium, copper, magnesium zinc, and potassium. Beans may play a role in decreasing incidents of colorectal cancer. Favored by people with diabetes, beans help reduce blood pressure and promote bone health.

Beets—Offering anti-inflammatory properties, beets are rich in phytonutrients such as folate, vitamin C, B6, iron, phosphorous, calcium, magnesium, niacin, thiamine, zinc, and riboflavin, plus they contain vulgaxanthin, an antioxidant. They also provide boron, a nutrient directly involved with the production of human sex hormones.

Bell Peppers—Fairly low in sugar and high in vitamin C, bell peppers contain a number of antioxidants such as alpha-carotene, beta-carotene, lycopene, zeaxanthin, lutein, and cryptoxanthin. Rely on the carotenoids for healthier eyes and to lower the risk of cardiovascular disease and cancer.

Blackberries—A good source of fiber, blackberries provide vitamin C, and are thought to address heart disease, urinary tract infections, and mental issues related to age. These berries are rich in antioxidants, such as anthocyanin, considered as having anti-cancer properties.

Blueberries—Similar in antioxidant and nutritional value as most other berries, blueberries, containing anti-inflammatory phytonutrients, are recommended for lowering cholesterol, slowing the process of aging, and lessening the risk of diabetes. A number of studies confirm blueberries support cardiovascular health.

Broccoli—Mom said to eat it, and she was right. A nutritional storehouse, broccoli is stuffed with antioxidants, vitamins, and beta-carotene as well as calcium, iron, selenium, and potassium. Recent research indicates the sulforaphane in broccoli may help breast cancer survivors remain cancer free, and broccoli's combination of antioxidants, anti-inflammatory, and detoxification abilities make this vegetable valuable in overall cancer prevention.

Brussels Sprouts—An anti-inflammatory, Brussels sprouts may help prevent heart disease and are loaded with omega-3 fatty acids (ALA), vitamins A and E, thiamine, niacin, and folate. Brussels sprouts have been the subject of more than one hundred scientific studies and half of those studies address this vegetable's anti-cancer benefits.

Cantaloupe—Slice open a cantaloupe to find vitamin C and a huge supply of beta-carotene. The carotenoids are a source of vitamin A.

Carrots—Vitamin A and beta-carotene make this garden vegetable a winner. Antioxidant properties provide numerous cardio-protective benefits, according to numerous medical studies worldwide.

Celery—A bit boring, but celery packs a punch, including phtalides, compounds known to lower cholesterol as well as blood pressure. It also contains vitamin C, beta-carotene, and manganese. The pectin-based polysaccharides may benefit the digestive system, especially the stomach.

Cherries—Iron, calcium, vitamins A and C make cherries a strong nutritional choice. In addition, they pack an antioxidant heart-healthy wallop. The melatonin found in tart cherries helps lower the body temperature and prepare the body for a restful sleep.

Chicken—Eaten without the skin, chicken breast is a low-fat protein high in niacin. Amino acids support cardiac health and skeletal muscles. This meat contains B vitamins, folate, biotin, and choline.

Edamame—Full of protein and nutrients, the green soy bean,

edamame, may have properties that protect the body from cancer, heart disease, and diabetes. Contains folate, potassium, vitamin K, phosphorus, and magnesium.

Grapefruit—Packed with vitamin C and a good source of fiber. Select pink grapefruit for the additional benefits of lycopene, including its anti-prostate cancer properties for men.

Kale—A good source of natural calcium, kale offers a number of vitamins critical for overall health. The nervous system benefits when we eat kale. Studied for its antioxidant, anti-inflammatory, and anti-cancer nutrients, kale offers concentrations of carotenoids and flavonoids, both powerful types of antioxidants.

Oranges—More than an outstanding source of vitamin C, oranges supply folate, antioxidants, and fiber. In animal studies, the herperidin molecule found in oranges has been proven to lower cholesterol and blood pressure.

Pomegranate—If looking for antioxidants, you can't go wrong with pomegranate, stuffed with folate, vitamins C and K, and dietary fiber. It's shown to benefit the heart and circulatory system as well as acting as an inhibitor of several cancers, including breast cancer, prostate cancer, and leukemia.

Quinoa—Among the most nutritious foods, protein-rich quinoa is an excellent source of manganese, phosphorus, and magnesium.

Raspberries—In addition to providing fiber and vitamin C, raspberries offer antioxidants that studies indicate address urinary tract infections, heart disease, and some cancers. They also have anthocyanins that promote good memory.

Salmon—Enjoy salmon for the taste and receive a boost of omega-3 fats and protein. We know that omega-3 is fundamental for healthy brain tissue and promotes strong hearts; however, the bioactive peptides may also support joint cartilage and help control inflammation in the digestive tract.

Sardines—A blue-ribbon source of omega-3, sardines are the little fish with big benefits, namely niacin, calcium, protein, vitamins D and B12, selenium, and phosphorous. Sardines promote heart health, bone health, and may play a role in preventing certain types of cancer.

Shiitake Mushrooms—Containing the compound lentinan, shiitake mushrooms yield anti-cancer agents, particularly for colorectal and stomach cancers. They strengthen the immune system and lower cholesterol, and have been known for thousands of years for their medicinal qualities.

Spinach—Popeye ate it, and so should you, because it's rich in antioxidants, natural calcium, and vitamin A. Protects against inflammatory conditions and cardiovascular problems while promoting bone health. May have anti-cancer benefits.

Strawberries—A good source of fiber and vitamin C, strawberries aid in stomach health and have been shown to slow the cognitive decline in the elderly. The fruit through research has been shown to be beneficial for cardiovascular support, blood sugar regulation, and prevention of cancer, particularly breast cancer, cervical cancer, and colon cancer.

Sweet Potatoes—Eat sweet potatoes to boost the immune system. Packed with vitamin A, beta-carotene, folate, potassium, and fiber, sweet potatoes improve the regulation of blood sugar.

Tomatoes—The cancer-fighter lycopene is only one attribute credited to tomatoes, respected for their vitamin C content and rich in antioxidants. Research indicates tomatoes reduce the risk of heart disease, promote bone health, and may offer anti-cancer properties.

Putting natural, whole foods in our bodies is the best way to take full advantage of the wonder that is our digestive system. This multifaceted part of our anatomy transforms nutrient-rich foods into the stuff of life, a body that loves movement and can perform amazing feats of strength and agility, a mind that reasons well beyond the capacity of any computer, while digestion of these super foods also fuels the body's system that gives pleasure, feels pleasure, and has the energy and will to fulfill any purpose.

"Love the body you received.
You only get one."
—Ashly

20:

We Are Made Perfectly Magnificent

At birth, our bodies are as perfect as they will ever be. The moment we take our first breath, we begin the process of aging, for most of us a gradual progression through childhood, adolescence, the various phases of adulthood, and inevitably, old age. We are barely out of the cradle when many of us are introduced to foods that do more harm than good: packaged breakfast cereals, sugar-rich cookies, soda containing the cane sugar substitute, high fructose corn syrup (HFCS), and fast food kid's meals of fried, salty potatoes and high-fat ground meat served between carbohydrate-rich white bread. Before entering kindergarten, many Americans are already craving a trash diet low in nutrients and high in sugar and saturated fat.

As wondrous as the digestive system of a newborn is, years of abuse can and will overwhelm it and that destruction does not take much time. The U.S. government has been keeping tabs. According to the Centers for Disease Control and Prevention, the average weight of teen boys in 1960 was 125 pounds; 118 pounds for girls. Today, the average teen boy tips the scale at 141 pounds; girls at 130 pounds. Incidence of obesity in teenagers has tripled in the past thirty years. Go into any high school in the early 1980s and, in a classroom of thirty kids, two children would be considered heavy. Today, in that school, the same classroom, at least ten of the teens are overweight or obese. A third of all American children and adolescents are carrying excess body fat. As adults, they will likely suffer from heart disease, prematurely age with osteoarthritis, and contract colon cancer, thyroid cancer, and any number of other ailments directly attributed to poor diet and weight gain.

The specialized organs, glands, and neurons comprising the digestive system face an overwhelming onslaught of crippling adversaries, most of our own choosing: chronic stress brought on by self-destructive thinking and the challenges inherent with coping in an unpredictable environment; lack of restful sleep; the use of prescribed and over-the-counter medications to treat symptoms of heartburn, irritable bowel syndrome (IBS) and similar ailments; exposure to heavy metals such as mercury; and the overuse of antibiotics that kill intestinal flora, the "good" bacteria living in the gut.

However, the most crippling adversary is a poor diet. For dinner, many Americans do not think twice about baking a frozen chicken pot pie loaded with salt and saturated fat or stopping at a chain restaurant and ordering the salt-and-fat soaked "Tour of Italy." Another chain eatery is famous for its cheesecake. Try the chocolate truffle that weighs close to a pound and contains as much fat as an entire stick of butter. There's the chain of coffee shops offering the twenty-ounce chocolate mochas and the fast food outlets peddling meals high in fats, salt, and unhealthy cholesterol. Our bodies were not designed to digest such trash. Here are the worst of the worst and why:

Manufactured Partially Hydrogenated Oil

A number of years ago, food preparers invented a way to considerably extend the shelf life of vegetable oils by adding hydrogen. The process, called hydrogenation, was a huge boon to the food industry and a big money maker. The idea of making manufactured products with hydrogenated trans fatty acids was an overnight success. In no time, grocery shelves and freezer displays were stocked with crackers, cakes, cookies, snacks, and frozen foods baked with these inexpensive, processed trans fats. Sticks and tubs of margarine and cans of shortening contained it. Fast food restaurants fried potato sticks and chicken pieces in trans fats and doughnut shops used it too.

Today, a number of manufacturers and restaurants have reduced the use of trans fats. Why? The human digestive system, unable to process this manmade ingredient, sent it into the bloodstream to clog and harden the arteries and generally wreak havoc. Are trans fatty acids a thing of the past? Hardly. Not yet outlawed in most places, trans fats continue to be prevalent in the food supply, particularly in manufactured frozen foods, frozen pie crusts, cake frostings, pancake mixes, and frozen fried chicken. Even if the product label lists no trans fats, that may not be the case. By law, if the product contains less than 0.5 grams of trans fats per serving, the label can read zero. To retain the crispiness or smoothness consumers expect of the products, manufacturers dilute the trans fats with vegetable oil or water to reduce the total amount per serving to under 0.5 grams.

Manufactured Sugar

Researchers at Louisiana State University, studying the nation's obesity epidemic, determined it paralleled the introduction of high-fructose corn syrup (HFCS) to the American diet. Between 1967 and 2000, the years when obesity took off to become prevalent, the consumption of HFCS increased 1000 percent, more than any other food or food group. Another study published in the Journal of the American Medical Association determined the consumption of soft drinks containing HFCS rose 86 percent between 1970 and 1997, while obesity increased 112 percent during the same approximate timeframe. Presently, HFCS is used as the primary sweetener in forty percent of the foods that have "manufactured sweeteners" and in all soft drinks.

In the digestive system, HFCS is metabolized as fructose, the sugar commonly found in fruits and some vegetables. As the small intestine processes the fructose derived from the consumption of fruits and vegetables, the amount of fructose, considered relatively minute, is gradually absorbed by the bloodstream. In contrast, the fructose level in HFCS is enormous. To counteract this spike in fructose sugar, the liver and pancreas go into overdrive, resulting in unnatural raging liver metabolism and pancreatic exhaustion.

In the overworking liver, some of this concentrated fructose, turned into glycogen, is stored for later use as a back-up source of energy, and when the liver soon reaches capacity to store more glycogen, it turns the fructose, which could be a considerable amount, into triglycerides, then converts this substance into lipoproteins, material that is stored in the fat cells. Often, there is so much fructose in the small intestine that a portion of it is sent on to the large intestine, introducing more disruption. Bacteria living in the large intestine love the sweet fructose. As a result of the feeding frenzy, the bacteria give off copious amounts of gases such as hydrogen, methane, carbon dioxide, and hydrogen sulfide. These fermented gases cause bloating, discomfort, and possibly constipation.

Manufactured Meats

They say about sausages that it's best not to see them made. As delicious as they are convenient, hot dogs, salami, bologna, bacon, ham, pepperoni, and hundreds of varieties of processed deli meats are at or near the top of any list of "the worst things to eat" and for good reason. The American Institute of Cancer Research pegged cured, salted, preservative-packed processed meats as a major contributor to colorectal cancer. In one study, researchers found that eating the equivalent of one-half hot dog a day increased the risk of colon cancer by a whopping forty-nine percent.

For a while, scientists suspected the primary culprit was the ubiquitous preservative, nitrate. Long ago, food makers discovered foods cured with sodium nitrate, a type of salt, resisted the bacteria that caused spoilage while helping the meat retain an appetizing color. In and of itself, sodium nitrate, a naturally occurring mineral, now appears to be harmless, since it is found in many vegetables. Nitrate has been debunked by a number of researchers as the culprit, leaving scientists to point to the high fat content of processed meats. A recent study tracked the eating habits of British, German, and Spanish meat eaters plus citizens of seven other European nations. Nearly half a million people participated in the study, which concluded that people who ate a lot of processed meats were more likely to die from heart failure, stroke, or cancer.

Despite the negative publicity buzzing around processed meats, Americans continue to eat them to the tune of more than $22 billion in retail sales and twenty billion hotdogs a year. It's estimated, on average, the American consumer eats more than two pounds of dogs, deli ham, and other processed meats every month. Researchers have yet to determine why processed meats likely target the digestive system and contribute to colorectal cancer.

Whether we are enjoying a deli-meat sandwich or a fried chicken dinner with a large soda, our meal is soon forgotten once we push away from the table, but the story of that meal's assimilation into the body is only getting started. Out of sight, out of mind, the body's digestive system kicks into high gear. A portion of the nutrients and sugars will be used to power your magnificent body, replenish cellular tissue, and make possible physiological functions we are only beginning to understand. Simultaneously, other parts of the meal are perpetrating mayhem and devastation on an unimaginable scale. We are born with a wondrous body. How we maintain it is up to each of us.

"When the mind and body are in balance, we digest our foods and our thoughts in a state of physical and emotional harmony."
—Ashly

21:

Sugar & Fat, a Complicated Relationship

As goes the digestive system, so goes our health. Although researchers and scientists have thoroughly studied the gastrointestinal system, there is much we do not know, and one area that continues to be debated is the relationship of insulin, cortisol, and the assimilation of sugars into glucose, the body's primary fuel source. Inside the pancreas, the endocrine gland secretes three critical hormones, insulin, glucagon, and somatostatin.

As sugars in the small intestine are converted into glucose, the pancreas, detecting the rise in glucose, sends the hormone insulin into the small intestine. Meeting with the glucose, the insulin helps move the glucose through the blood stream to every cell in the body requiring energy to function. In a delicate balancing act, somatostatin determines the exact amount of insulin needed to make sure the cells receive enough glucose for energy, but not enough to be overwhelmed. Assisted by insulin, some of the glucose, diverted from cell usage, is temporarily stored in the liver as the substance glycogen. By the way, when the liver is filled with glycogen, excess glycogen is changed into triglycerides for longer-term storage in the fat cells.

If the body misses a meal or requires a quick burst of energy, glucose energy is suddenly required. For example, we decide to go from a casual walk to an all-out run, lift weights, or jump for joy. As glucose in cells rapidly depletes, the pancreas immediately secretes glucagon, and then sends this hormone to the liver to convert the stored glycogen into glucose, which pours into the blood stream, replenishing the cells that need more energy.

When everything is working in harmony, life's good. For reasons not well understood by physicians and researchers, a person can overproduce such large amounts of insulin that the body can no longer use it. This is called insulin resistance. On the other hand, the pancreas can slow or stop making insulin altogether. Both conditions result in type 2 diabetes. Either way, sugar glucose builds to extreme levels in the bloodstream until the person's brain will dysfunction, resulting in coma, and even death.

Individuals with type 2 diabetes must take careful readings of their blood sugar levels once a day or several times a week, monitor the foods and portion sizes they eat, exercise, and perhaps use medications or receive insulin injections.

Those carrying excessive weight and physically inactive are prone to this condition, but there are instances of thin people getting type 2 diabetes and cases of heavy people never getting it. Experts tell us, it's possible that genetics may play a role, but type 2 diabetes continues to rise along with the nation's obesity rate. The dramatic increase in obesity in the United States since 1990, with a third of the population now considered obese, matches the number of people with type 2 diabetes. The highest rates of both obesity and type 2 diabetes are in the same places: the Appalachian region of Kentucky, Tennessee, and West Virginia; and in the southern states of Alabama, Georgia, Louisiana, Mississippi, and South Carolina. According to the Centers for Disease Control and Prevention, 81 percent of Appalachian counties have the highest rates of incidence of both obesity and type 2 diabetes, and 77 percent of the counties in the South.

Every year, diabetes contributes to more than 200,000

American deaths, according to the American Diabetes Association, and thousands of new cases of heart disease and stroke, hypertension, blindness, kidney disease, nervous system damage, and amputations.

For some people who are morbidly obese, losing the weight does not necessarily restore the pancreas' ability to again secrete insulin. However, if the pancreas is not damaged beyond repair, type 2 diabetes can be partially, and, in rare instances, fully reversed to the point where medications are no longer needed. Most success cases involve individuals with less severe or newly diagnosed type 2 diabetes.

Assuming our pancreas is harmoniously pumping out correct amounts of insulin, glucagon, and somatostatin, we have three stress hormones, all secreted by the adrenal gland. Adrenalin, norepinephrine, and cortisol are designed to keep us safe, secure, and out of danger. Of the three, the hormone adrenaline is the "fight or flight" substance. Imagine you're enjoying a hiking trail along the rim of an Arizona canyon, taking in incredible vistas, when, out of the corner of your eye, you see movement under a yucca plant. Investigating, you come face-to-face with a diamondback rattlesnake, coiled and about to strike. You take off running in the opposite direction, sprinting hard, your heart pounding, perspiration pouring out, and your breathing ragged. That's adrenaline coming to your rescue. Adrenaline, instantly putting the body in high gear, channels every fiber of your being to either fight or take flight.

Getting your breathing and heart rate under control, you continue to jog away from the canyon rim, intent on putting distance between you and the rattler. The senses are on high alert as you scan the trail ahead of you. No detail goes unnoticed, the shadow of a rock, the movement of some dust, anything that could indicate danger. This is norepinephrine doing its job. This hormone heightens awareness and focuses our senses and mind on the task at hand, which, in this case, is avoiding more snakes.

Later, back in the comfort of your hotel room, you think about what could have been. You fret about the possibility of again encountering a snake, worry about the consequences of a venomous bite that could paralyze and kill. The more you turn the events of the day over in your mind, reliving every second of the encounter, fear rises from deep within. Blood pressure spikes, anxiety grabs hold, and panic threatens to overpower the senses. These are the effects of cortisol, the stress hormone.

Angry over an argument with a friend, upset about your job, stuck in traffic and late for an appointment, having something on your mind and not able to sleep, or stressed about losing weight, these states are all sources of anxiety, and, when we are anxious, we produce cortisol. Potentially powerful, cortisol-driven anxiety, if it becomes chronic, elevates blood pressure, decreases libido, and increases levels of glucose in the blood. In this heightened state of apprehension, cortisol may inhibit insulin, forcing the liver to make excess triglycerides that find their way to fat cell storage. In and of itself, cortisol does not make anyone fat; however, a long-term, higher-than-normal level of cortisol is suspected of amplifying the storage of sugars already present in the digestive system. These excess triglycerides end up in the belly fat cells. That's why practicing meditation techniques such as yoga to reduce stress may be helpful in keeping extra triglycerides out of the fat cells.

That brings us to processing fat and fat storage, some of the least understood functions of the human body. In a broad sense, fat is where the body turns to for energy when food is not immediately available, such as when we skip a meal or begin eating appreciably less. Science investigators did not give fat much thought until 1994, when researchers discovered fat secreted a hormone, leptin, which tended to inhibit appetite. Since then, scientists have uncovered several other hormones, all secreted by fat or the fat cells, that may work in the body to address inflammations, protect against type 2 diabetes, and play various roles in controlling metabolism.

Scientists at Boston University's Diabetes and Nutrition Research Center, Harvard Medical School, and the Kaiser Permanente Division of Research in Oakland, California, have taken intense interest in this stuff that seems to plague our midsections and hips. They tell us all fat is not the same. It turns out we carry four types of fat in varying amounts and degrees: brown fat; white fat; subcutaneous fat; and visceral fat, commonly thought of as belly fat. Fat is stored in "fat cells," and we have more or less the same number of fat cells in our body; however, these cells are highly elastic, able to expand many times larger than their original size.

Brown Fat

We're not sure why people have brown fat, but in some ways, it acts more like a muscle than the other kinds of fat and, when the temperature drops, it tends to use white fat as a source of energy. Brown fat, much more prevalent in children, may have been nature's way to keep youngsters warm on cold nights in the prehistoric cave. As we age, we lose brown fat, but, comparatively speaking, we don't have that much to begin with. If a woman weighs 150 pounds, twenty to thirty pounds of that weight can be attributed to fat, and only three ounces of that is in brown fat. However, that tiny bit of brown fat is dispersed throughout the body. For reasons we do not comprehend, leaner individuals carry more brown fat than their heavier counterparts. Due to brown fat's ability to "burn" white fat to keep the body warm, some people residing in northern climates suggest leaving the bedroom window open on winter nights. They claim to lose a pound a week as a form of weight loss.

White Fat

Just under the skin and dispersed throughout the body, white fat stores energy. White fat can secrete adiponectin, a hormone that interacts with insulin and plays a role in storing energy and removing it when needed. White fat, serving as a blanket of insulation, helps keep our body temperature where it needs to be.

Subcutaneous Fat

This is the fat found directly under the skin's white fat layer. We measure subcutaneous fat with calipers to help determine overall fitness and estimate one's total body fat. Thought of as important in cushioning the body, subcutaneous fat in the thighs and buttocks areas is necessary for comfort. However, in the mid section, subcutaneous fat may enhance belly fat.

Visceral Fat

If you have a "muffin top," large waist measurement, and big belly, your internal organs are enveloped in visceral fat, the so-called "deep fat" that is the most troublesome for health and a long life. Initially, this deep fat attaches to the lining of the abdominal cavity and surrounds the major organs such as the liver, heart, kidneys, and intestines, then, at the stomach, especially for men, forms a hanging flap over the intestinal area, while in women, it enlarges the hips, upper thighs, buttocks, and breasts. Many people with large quantities of visceral fat are candidates for type 2 diabetes, heart disease and stroke, ovarian cystic disease, breast cancer, and sleep apnea.

Visceral fat presses on the organs, diminishing their effectiveness, and places an inordinate strain on hip and knee joints. In the extreme, visceral fat will hamper the ability to maintain a proper posture, eventually relegating the person to a wheelchair.

The rotund appearance known as belly fat is actually a combination of the surface level subcutaneous fat and the visceral fat underneath. These two types of fat become so entwined, a CT scan is required to tell where one ends and the other stops. At first, men tend to gain "belly fat" in the midsection, while women more commonly store fat in the breasts, hips, and buttocks.

In the process of losing weight, the removal of fat to convert to energy, the body initially targets visceral fat. To see how much, a research scientist at Duke University Medical Center, Chris Slentz, conducted an eight-month study of middle-aged men and women, having one group briskly walk thirty minutes a day, six days a week; a second group jog instead of walk; and a third group do nothing. The walkers carried the same amount of visceral fat at the end of the study, the joggers had a noticeable reduction in fat, and the group that did not exercise saw an increase of 8.6 percent in visceral fat.

Working with several obese men and women as clients, I have concluded it is best to introduce change gradually by altering their eating habits, offering healthier food choices, and encouraging moderate exercise. As a man, you will not go from wearing a 52-inch belt to a 38-inch one, and a woman to having a 34-inch waist, overnight. Ten, twenty, or more years of growing girth will not be reversed in a matter of months; but, in time, it can be done.

I have mentioned the hormone leptin, the substance secreted in fat cells that tells the brain we are full. Research indicates the profoundly obese can become "leptin-resistant," meaning the brain ignores the hormone's signal to stop eating. An opposite hormone, produced in the stomach lining as well as in the pancreas, ghrelin, discovered in the late 1990s, signals when we are hungry. Think of grehlin as the gremlin that makes noise in the tummy when it's empty. In a way, grehlin is our short-term body weight regulator telling us it's time to eat.

Since about twenty to thirty minutes are required for the stomach gremlin to quiet again, it's a good idea to slow your eating. Gobbling down the meal in a matter of a few minutes short circuits the grehlin signal, causing you to continue feeling hungry, and become likely to eat more. In addition, the grehlin gremlin is thought to increase our cravings for sugary, high-fat foods. Some studies suggest when we are sleep-deprived, ghrelin production significantly increases, possibly explaining why some people who awake in the night raid the pantry for sugary treats such as ice cream and cookies.

To keep leptin-resistance and the ghrelin gremlin levels in check, and our eating in balance, I suggest starting the day with a high-fiber breakfast of oatmeal or quinoa; organic, sprouted whole grain Ezekiel bread with nut butter; eggs; or a protein smoothie made of fruit and a cup of greens. For a snack, try fruits or veggies.

At lunchtime, keep it simple and take a full half-hour. Keep favorites on hand for an easy-to-prepare meal, such as a chicken lettuce wrap or green salad with chicken, mushrooms, and olive oil dressing. Consider a mid-afternoon snack that's high in essential fatty acids, thought to act on leptin production that tells us we are full. A snack high in essential fatty acids would be nuts and seeds, fresh coconut, or avocado.

Don't skip dinner. Doing so gets the gremlin growling, making sugary foods and carbs, like dinner rolls, that much more inviting. Enjoy a meal of lean protein and fresh vegetables, such as my favorites, butternut or spaghetti squash. Squash is nutritious and gives you a satisfied feeling.

At all meals, be seated at a table. Relax, possibly listen to music, and enjoy the pleasure of the dining experience.

Eating and digesting well is not a matter of willpower, rather it is a matter of mindfulness. We love and embrace our body to the point where we want to treasure it, and nourish it with wholesome foods and the movement it desires. When the mind and body are in balance, we digest our foods and our thoughts in a state of physical and emotional harmony. Do these things, and you are in the **END Zone**.

"Physically and soulfully embrace your body. Nourish it with food, movement, and rest. Digest your food, thoughts, and emotions in harmony as nature intended."
—Ashly

22:

Honor the Body, Honor the Dream

Emily was a member of my ten-week "boot camp," a gathering of women and a few men interested in improving fitness through movement and nutrition. Her goal was to lose fifteen pounds, build muscle, and improve metabolism. On the camp's last day, she was radiant. "I have more energy than I've had in a long time," she told me, flashing an enthusiastic smile. "I'm eating better foods, stretching before bedtime, and I'm not getting cravings for sugary snacks in the afternoons and evenings like I did. I'm mindful about what I eat, how I eat, and I'm loving my new self."

Another member of a boot camp class, Claire, sent me an email. "I wanted to share some things that happened since going to your classes," she wrote. "I had chronic knee pain when I crouched to load and unload the washer and dryer. The pain is gone and so are my other regular aches and pains. I'm no longer winded going up the stairs. I have more energy. My legs and thighs feel much tighter (noticeably, when I lotion them), and my nails are growing. Could that be the increased oxygen in my system?"

In a note, Trish told me, "I can now stretch and touch my toes. Never have been able to do that! Sleeping through the night, playing tennis, and there's no pain. You sure improved my quality of life."

No, Trish, you improved your quality of life by embracing your wonderful body, providing the nourishment it needed, and digesting your foods and thoughts in a state of harmony and relaxation.

Through another boot camp participant, I met Addie. "I've heard about your classes," she said, during that first phone conversation. "My friend, Janice, told me how you really helped turn her life around. I can't come to your next boot camp, but will you take me on as a client? Before you answer, I'll warn you, you'll have your work cut out for you."

Two days later, in the doorway of a spare office at a YMCA, stood Addie, nervous and apprehensive. Taking a seat on the couch, she avoided looking directly at me, fidgeted with the leather wristband of her watch, and may have bolted, if I had not taken her hand.

"I hope you don't mind," I gently said. "We only have met, but I think you need a friend, someone who will listen. Is it okay if I hold your hand for a moment?"

For the first time, she fixed her eyes on mine and nodded.

"Addie, let's begin by your telling me a little about yourself? Would that be okay?"

Nodding again, Addie spoke in a timid, but clear voice. She was twenty-nine, employed at a finance company, and not married. "I've always loved food, and my parents did, too. I was the only girl in a family with three brothers, and I was the baby. My dad gave me sweets all the time. I was this plump little girl, loving the attention, eating candy, cookies, cake, and ice cream, and it didn't help that I preferred playing house with my dolls instead of kicking a ball or riding bikes with my brothers. In college, I weighed over two-hundred pounds, and, after college, I continued to gain weight. Everyone said I was fun and bubbly, but inside, I was embarrassed and ashamed. I guess you could say I learned to put on a happy face. At the office, I'm the one who brings cookies or brownies on Fridays, and I end up eating half of them myself."

Tears stained her cheeks. I gave her a tissue, and she continued. "I've had dates, but I've never had a boyfriend, and it was really hard for me to finally get a job. When I'm alone and unhappy, I eat, especially sweets. Believe me, I know all about comfort food."

Detecting a slight smile cross her lips, I ventured, "So, what has changed?"

"Janice was raving about you at the office. How you helped her think about her life in a new way, to eat better and take care of herself," Addie replied. "I went back to my desk and I can't really explain it, but I came to the realization that I have to change my life. I don't want to live this way anymore. I asked Janice for your number, and here I am. I warned you when I called," she quickly added. "You have your work cut out for you. I weighed myself this morning. I'm 269 pounds."

"That's the first thing we're going to do," I said with a smile.

"What's that?"

"Get rid of that scale, because you won't need it anymore."

"I like you already," Addie laughed. It was the start of a friendship and client relationship I still treasure.

In the days that followed, I invited Addie to join me in the **END Zone**.

The first assignment was to write a letter from her body. Here is the letter:

Dear Addie,

For so many years, you did not listen to my needs, feed me good things, or take care of me. I've worked hard to be there for you, never complaining, but it hurt me not to have you love me as much as I love you. I know that all of those sugary treats made you feel better, but they were very damaging to me. As much as I wanted you to be comforted, it was at my expense. I'm glad you asked Ashly for help, because I don't think I could have gone on much longer. My legs hurt, my joints creak, and I'm tired of carrying all this extra weight. Please change your ways. Please pay attention to me. Please love me.

These letters are usually very personal and may be kept private. However, Addie gave it to me to read and share, and this heartfelt message brought me to tears. Later, I learned she framed the letter, along with a photo of herself, as a reminder to embrace and love her body.

"Do you like your work?" I inquired during one of our initial sessions. "Do you enjoy what you do at the finance company?"

"Pretty much," Addie said. "It's fun to help a young couple buy their first house, but that's not what I want to do for the rest of my life."

"Tell me," I pressed. "What would be your dream job?"

"I'd like to go for my MBA, become a financial planner, and help people with their investments, so they can send their kids to college and have a secure retirement."

"That's a wonderful career ambition," I noted. "I think you would be very good at doing that, because you're goal-oriented and care about people." Smiling, I followed up with another question. "Is there anything you have always wanted to do? Anywhere you want to travel, perhaps?"

"Actually, there is," Addie answered as she brightened. "When I was a kid, I had this picture book about the Fiji Islands. If I could do anything, I'd go to Fiji, stay in one of those huts over the water, and swim with the tropical fish."

Later that week, I purchased a book and gave it to my new client. It was an oversized, coffee table book illustrated with gorgeous color photography depicting the romance of the Pacific Islands, particularly the islands of Fiji. Inscribing the book, I wrote, "We honor our bodies, so we can honor our dreams!"

Gradually, Addie purged her kitchen of carbohydrate-rich convenience foods, replacing frozen pizzas, pot pies, and ready-made pasta dinners with fresh salad greens, vegetables, fruits, chicken breast, and seafood, such as salmon. At the office and at home, we substituted water and green tea for her six-pack-of-cola-a-day habit. To avoid caffeine withdrawal, Addie took two months to stop drinking soda, but she did it.

While eliminating unhealthy foods from her kitchen, we talked about abolishing toxic thoughts and beliefs from her mind. What were some of these toxic beliefs? Sweets bring comfort. Fitness is an impossibility. Lack of success is about lack of willpower. "Stay present with your authentic self," I suggested. "When a toxic, negative belief seeps into your mind, take time to banish it." We talked about sorting truth from the fictional beliefs that unnecessarily burden us with mental baggage.

Does it resonate true?

Is it unquestionably true?

How do you feel when you believe it is true?

How would you visualize yourself, if that idea never entered your mind to begin with?

What affirmation comes to mind at this moment?

We practiced meditation, breathing, and talked about slowing down to be mindful at mealtimes. Reflecting her background in finance, Addie was committed to keeping daily logs, conscientiously recording what and when she ate and her exercise routines. On a number of occasions, rather than meeting at the YMCA or a health club, we walked the trails of a metro park, taking in the beauty of a lake, a canopy of oak trees, and other pleasures of the natural world.

It was not always idyllic work for Addie. Often, her sugar cravings were enormous. "Go ahead, buy a chocolate pie once every two weeks," I counseled. "But buy the very best chocolate pie you can find, then cut a slice and eat it slowly, mindfully, relishing every ounce of flavor and texture. Satisfy the craving, and then throw the rest of the pie away."

"If I get started, I'll eat the whole thing," she fretted.

"Maybe, and maybe not," I replied, urging her to give it a try. "I think you'll be pleasantly surprised. Once you satisfy the craving by giving yourself the very best, and eating it purposefully, it will be more than enough."

When we met again, Addie was ecstatic. "You were right," she responded, beaming. "In fact, I couldn't eat the entire slice of pie. I was satisfied."

"In the **END Zone**, we don't believe in denying our cravings," I explained. "But when we eat to fulfill our purpose, the cravings pale in comparison."

Following various meal plans created for her, exercising on a daily basis, and applying a number of yoga and breathing techniques, Addie was able to purchase a smaller dress size.

About six months and several progressively smaller dress sizes after our first get-acquainted meeting in that YMCA spare office, Addie and I were talking. "How much do you think I should weigh?" she questioned.

"That's up to you, but it's not necessarily about weight," I countered. "The question we need to consider is, 'What is the ideal level of fitness for you?'"

"What is my ideal level of fitness?" she responded, confusion in her voice.

"To fulfill your purpose, what shape, physically and mentally, would be ideal for you?"

"I don't know."

"You want to earn your MBA and become a financial planner, right?"

"Yes, that's my career goal."

"How about traveling to Fiji and swimming with the tropical fish?"

"I'm doing it, someday."

"Then, that's your ideal level of fitness," I clarified. "Let's help you gain the strength, vigor, and stamina you need to return to college, become a financial planner, and scuba dive in the waters of your Pacific paradise."

"Live for my purpose, right?"

"Absolutely," I affirmed. "Eat like the person you want to become. Exercise your body to enjoy your best life. Reshape your attitudes and beliefs, and in the process, reshape the future to fulfill your dreams."

"Guess what?" Addie practically screamed. Nearly a year had passed since we started working together. "What?" I replied, nearly as loud to match her enthusiasm.

"I've joined a scuba club."

"Wow! Tell me about it."

"It's right here in the city," she enthused. "They offer lessons at a pool, and once you're certified, you can go on dive trips to practice your skills. We fly as a group, and they go to amazing places. Last month's dive trip was to Key Largo, and the next trip, in about three months, is to Costa Rica. But the amazing thing is, hold on to your hat, in six months, we're going to the Beqa Lagoon Resort in Fiji. Can you believe it?" Then she repeated, more enthusiastic than before, "Can you believe it?"

"So, you're going."

"I've signed up for the lessons," she replied and grinned from ear to ear. "The Fiji dates are in my planner. You bet. I'll be there!"

What a difference a year can make.

Addie learned to scuba dive, joined the South Seas dive trip, and continues to replace her wardrobe with smaller dresses. She is now a size six. She has been dating another dive club member, and recently completed her first semester at the university to earn the MBA she coveted.

A frequent member of my three-day-a-week boot camp, Addie was speaking with a first-timer to the class. Passing by, I heard my client and friend offer the advice: "It's best to schedule regular times for exercise and movement, eat the foods your body needs and, most of all, know what you want. By the way, get rid of the scale. You don't need it anymore. You see, we honor our bodies, so we can honor our dreams."

Smiling, I started the class with a fun movement routine.

PART 4:

TOOLS FOR
HEALTHIER LIVING

*"To maximize the **END Zone** health and fitness advantage, we need specialized tools that help us embrace, nourish and digest."*
—*Ashly*

Just as a carpenter reaches into a box of tools for the right device to complete a job, in the **END Zone**, we have a number of specialized tools to help us fashion a healthier lifestyle. For mind, heart, and body, here are "go-to" tools you can use right away.

TOOL NO. 1: Awaken the Mind
TOOL NO. 2: Fill Up with Affirmations
TOOL NO. 3: One-Minute Movement Starters
TOOL NO. 4: The 30-Minute Workout

Basic Core and Advanced Level Workouts Instructions

TOOL NO. 5: Basic Core Routine 1
TOOL NO. 6: Basic Core Routine 2
TOOL NO. 7: Moderate Routine
TOOL NO. 8: Advanced Routine 1
TOOL NO. 9: Advanced Routine 2

TOOL NO. 10: Back Health & Maintenance
TOOL NO. 11: The Truth about Supplements
TOOL NO. 12: Successful Grocery Shopping
TOOL NO. 13: Quick & Easy Dinner Recipes

TOOL NO. 1:

Awaken the Mind

In the **END Zone**, mindfulness starts with an acute awareness of our bodies, the power of our thoughts, and a focused realization of our purpose in life. The act of using the diaphragm to draw oxygen deep into the lungs awakens the senses like nothing else. Several times a day, when we pause for a mindful moment to fill the body with oxygen, we inherently enter a tranquil state, slow the pace, and heighten awareness of ourselves and the environment around us. Similar to meditation, awakening the mind through deep breathing results in a form of harmony and equilibrium that prepares us for what's next, whether it be work or play. We perform at our best when deep breathing releases toxins and oxygenates our cellular tissues, soothes tension and brings clarity, and relieves muscle tension while enhancing our stamina. Heralded by physicians for hundreds of years, deep breathing is a technique anyone can master.

Taking in a deep breath through the nostrils, expand the chest into the lowest reaches of the abdomen. Hold the breath for a moment and then exhale. Gradually breathe in, hold, and exhale. Repeat three more times. As you breathe, feel the air in the lungs and imagine the oxygen traveling through the bloodstream to the brain, heart, and every fiber of your being. Slow and measured breathing calms the mind, boosts the immune system, increases digestion, and strengthens the heart, lungs, and other organs.

During the day, especially after lunch, our minds and bodies tend to become sluggish. It may not be convenient to stop and nap, so here are some reinvigoration strategies:

Body Rocks—Awaken the mind and body with a simple movement. On a floor mat, take a position on your back, hug the knees tightly into the chest, and rock back and forth from shoulders to lower back. This action stimulates cranial sacral fluids circulation in a way that energizes and rejuvenates mind and body. Try for sixty seconds. Over time, increase as desired.

Peppermint Essential Oil—One of my favorite oil scents, especially in the afternoon, peppermint oil stimulates my mind to become more aware and alert. Diffuse in an essential oil diffuser or apply a drop to the palm of the hand. Rub the palms in a circular motion, and then bring the palms to the nostrils. Breathe in the fragrance.

Mindful Walking—A type of meditation best done in nature, mindful walking reduces stress, lowers anxiety, and gets you in touch with mind and body. I suggest a minimum of ten minutes. As you walk, heighten your awareness of the natural world by enveloping your senses, stimulating the imagination, and paying attention to details, such as a bird's song, the breeze in the leaves of a tree, and grass under your feet. Before starting, some people close their eyes, take deep breaths, and attempt to become one with the world around them. I take a moment to be thankful for my life and the simple wonder of breathing. Upon opening my eyes, I take the initial steps in forcing myself to be aware of my body's movement, the contractions of the leg muscles, the placement of my feet on the path, and the swing of my arms. Next, I tune in my mind to capture all that I see, hear, and feel: the leaves on the trees, the sound of insects in the wind, and the warmth of the sun on my face. I notice details I would never have recognized, and I become one with the world around me. If troublesome thoughts enter your mind or you recall your "to-do" list, expunge them by centering your focus on your breathing, walking, and environment. With conscientious practice, you will learn to find a sense of inner peace you may not have yet experienced.

Keep a Journal—Clear the mind with paper, pen, and your thoughts. Journaling helps to release toxic views, organize one's thinking, and possibly identify troublesome issues. Whether you write in a notebook or use an iPad, start by taking several deep breaths to center and focus. Write whatever comes to mind. Unconcerned with grammar or sentence structure, release what's in your heart. It may be anger, fear, or frustration. Often the final few sentences reflect the truth of the matter and may suggest solutions such as the need to understand another's motives or be gracious in reaction to someone's actions.

Take Stock—Repeat the good, trash the not so good. A form of self-analysis, taking stock means objectively looking at your life to determine the people, actions and behaviors that energize you and those that drain your energy. Are there people in your life who make you feel energized and motivated? A style of music, a particular genre of reading, a type of exercise, a favorite approach to meditation, or any number of activities can be your "hot buttons" that get you up, stimulate the senses, and move you. When it comes to good people and good things, engage and repeat. In contrast, there may be people who are the first to complain, find fault in nearly everything and everybody, and rarely offer constructive ideas for improvement. Excessive drinking of alcoholic beverages dulls the senses. Wallowing in self-pity, hanging on to anger, and any number of other destructive behaviors sap energy. Be wary of negative people and beware of harmful activities.

Healthy Frivolity—Children value playfulness. So should we. Never grow up to the point where the child in you disappears. Our heart thrives on laughter, fun, and merriment. Awaken the mind and body with a good belly laugh.

Get in the Rhythm—We operate in a natural circadian

rhythm, synchronized with the twenty-four-hour cycle of the earth's rotation. If possible, match your lifestyle with the days of your lives. Awaken with the dawn, sleep after sunset. Consume the largest meal at midday, rely on deep breathing, a light snack of fruit or vegetables, and lots of water to get you through the afternoon, and eat a moderate-sized meal at the dinner hour. Avoid eating late, so your body can "take out the trash" and renew itself for the day to come. Get in rhythm, and you'll feel the difference like night and day.

Soulfully Focus—Try prayer and have a grateful heart. When we are grateful to have the body God gave us, the love of family and friends, and the unlimited bounty of this green earth, how can we not be joyous?

TOOL NO. 2:

Fill Up with Affirmations

A positive thought life requires a healthy dosage of affirmative thinking every day. Here are a number of reflections designed to fuel your optimism. Copy the ones that resonate with you on index cards. Tape them to your bathroom mirror as daily reminders to change your focus to affirm yourself. Take time to fill up with hopefulness.

On Prosperity:
I am prepared and open to receive blessings.
Everything always works out for me.
Everything that I do prospers.
I welcome abundance.
All that I need is always provided. I am at peace.
What I focus on with thought and feeling is what I attract.
All that is good and honorable comes my way.
I attract all that brings prosperity and abundance.
I choose to focus on the limitless possibilities that are my future.
I am the living, breathing example of my goal.
The choices I make today build my future.

I alone have the power to choose which possibility becomes reality in my life. I choose wisely.

On Daily Living:
Truth doesn't change.

I do my absolute best in everything every day.

Actions follow beliefs. What you believe is what will follow.

I am at peace, I am calm, and all is well.

No matter what occurs, all is right in my life and my world.

I am strong, confident and calm within.

I embrace the moment with openness.

I embrace uncertainty with a tranquil spirit and a warm heart.

As I release that which holds me down, the new, fresh and vital enters. Life flows through me with ease.

I have time and space for all that I need to do. I am at peace.

I embrace the beauty of today and all that it brings.

Today, I choose freedom from the chains that bind me.

I choose love for it empowers me.

I choose peace for it brings me calm.

I choose joy for it brings me passion.

I appreciate the variety and nuances of today's experiences.

I choose LIFE.

I express myself with love and truth.

Only good happens in my life, because I think, act and feel with love and truth.

It is not what you do; it is how you do it.

Life brings fantastic surprises!

I embrace the life that is before me.

I trust that no matter what, I am okay.

I only speak words of encouragement.

On Physical Fitness:
Weight loss is about living at your natural weight in a fun, pleasurable and love-filled way.

It is important to be healthy and approve of yourself, rather than thin and fittin' in.

I love and embrace my body as it is today and as it will be tomorrow.

My body is strong, mobile and flexible.

I live intentionally and will succeed in caring for my body and soul.

I choose to embrace, nourish, and digest food and life with ease, compassion and honor.

I honor this beautiful vessel that houses my soul and spirit.

I nourish myself with food that honors the intentions I have for my life and my body.

As I tune into my body, I discover messages that have been lying dormant.

Pain is a symptom with a divine message; I am open to discovering what it is and how it plays a role in my life.

I am safe.

I release the need for excess weight. I am worthy of a fit and healthy body.

I nourish my body and soul with nourishing food, so that I may live with enthusiasm and energy.

I choose to heal.

On the Soul & Spirit:
I am thankful for….

I surrender and am open to receive guidance and inspiration from my God.

Joy, peace and love flow through my mind, body and experiences.

I enfold myself and others in grace.

I love and I am loved by a love greater than what I could ever imagine.

I digest and assimilate food and life with ease.

Love and compassion radiate from me and into others.

I embrace uncertainty with openness.
I am a spirit of love, power, and self-discipline.
I am FREE to be ME.
I practice faith in everything.
I see each moment as a miracle.
I operate from my heart, so I may seek God's heart.
I am beautiful, just as I am.
I choose to forgive, release, and relax.
I live free, animated and motivated by God's spirit.
I am thankful for all I am learning and my beautiful life.

TOOL NO. 3:

One-Minute Movement Starters

The journey to fitness and a healthier lifestyle begins with the first step. For a "fresh start" to getting fit, consider one-minute movement breaks. Each one is a step in the right direction, bringing you from a sedentary lifestyle to an active one in no time. Success and sustainability begin with one step, one minute, and one movement. Each hour of your day, take a one-minute movement break to become more mobile and flexible. As a bonus, you will improve clarity of thought. Before starting any exercise program, consult your physician.

Basic

March in Place:

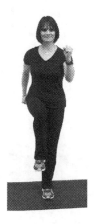 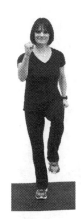

Bring knees to hip height. Repeat for one minute.

Low Impact Jumping Jacks:

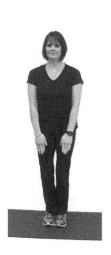 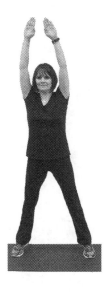

Step one foot out to your side at a time. Repeat for one minute.

Hand to Foot:

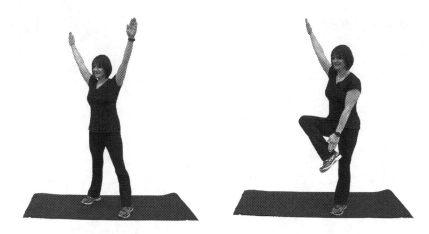

Stand with arms stretched overhead. Reach down with left arm and bring the right foot up to meet it in front of body. Alternate for one minute.

Cardio Hopscotch:

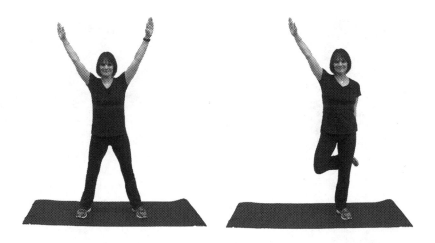

Stand with arms stretched overhead. Reach back with left arm and curl right leg behind to meet hand. Alternate sides for one minute.

Moderate

Standard Jumping Jacks:

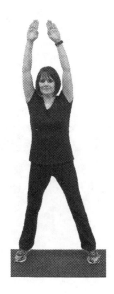

Keep abs tight to support the body. Repeat for one minute.

Cardio Seal Jacks:

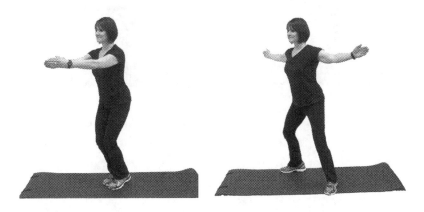

Same as Jumping Jacks, but arms come across the front of your body. Repeat for one minute.

Power Skate:

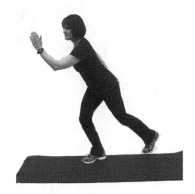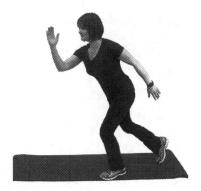

Leap from left to right. Keep chest and head up, abs in. Repeat for one minute.

In-Place Skip:

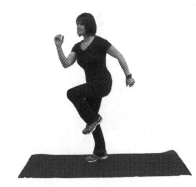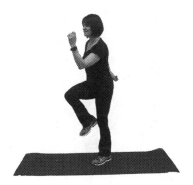

Relive childhood memories with the in-place skip! Skip in place just as you would skip down the street. Keep moving at a high intensity for one minute.

Advanced

Floor Jacks:

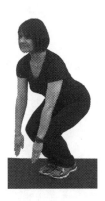 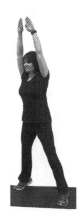

Begin with the feet together in a narrow squat position. Keep abs pulled in tight, shoulders back, face forward (NOT DOWN). Arms are extended to the ground. Power up and open legs into an inverted-V stance with the arms extended to the sky. Bring the legs back to a narrow stance and squat with the arms reaching to ground. Repeat for one minute.

Power Jacks:

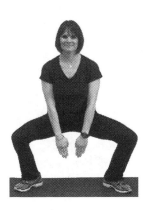 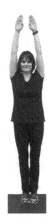

Begin in a wide squat with the hips low. Power up and bring feet together as arms reach overhead. Jump back up, land in a wide squat position, and bring arms down to center to complete the exercise. Repeat for one minute.

Skater Jumps:

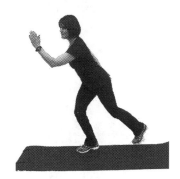 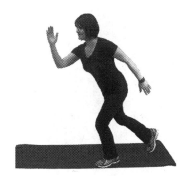

Jump side-to-side in a speed skater stance. Look straight ahead, shoulders back, abs in. Repeat for one minute.

Cardio Bench Hops:

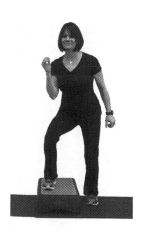 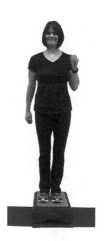

Hop over bench, alternating right and left foot on bench. Repeat for one minute.

Climb Stairs or Step-Ups on Bench:

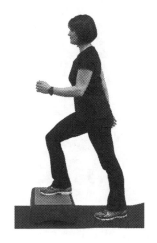
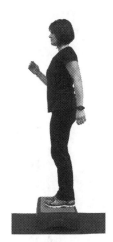

Climb stairs or alternate steps on a step bench. Repeat for one minute.

Cross the River:

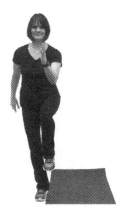
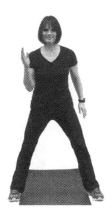
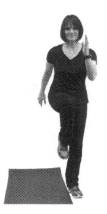

Leap side-to-side over a small or imaginary object. Repeat for one minute.

TOOL NO. 4:

The 30-Minute Workout

Meant for moderate fitness levels, the 30-Minute Workout includes four segments: warm up, strengthening, core and cardio, plus a cool-down. Follow the instructions listed for each segment. Before starting any exercise program, consult your physician.

Segment 1: Warm Up

Perform each exercise for 30 seconds or 15 repetitions (choose what works best for you). Repeat the circuit for five minutes.

Prisoner Body Weight Squat

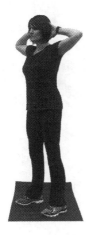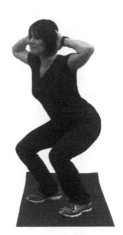

Hands behind head, medium stance, keeping shoulders back and chest upright, lower body until hips are at knee height. For more advanced, lower body as close to ground as possible. Drive heels into ground as you stand, squeeze the glutes.

High Knee March

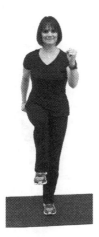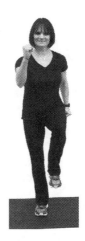

March in place, bringing knees up to hip level. Use big arm movements; pump them to shoulder height.

Power Front Kicks

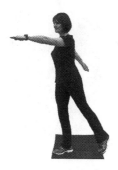 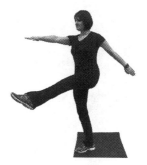

From the starting position, right leg extended behind, power kick leg forward. Maintain tight abs and kegel to support torso. Perform exercise on alternating left and right sides.

Segment 2: Strengthening

Perform each exercise in three sets of 20 repetitions. Repeat the circuit for 15 minutes.

Standing Chest Press with Tubing

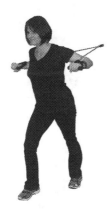 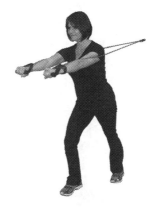

Insert tubing in middle of door hinge. Take hold of handles and face away from door. In relaxed position, elbows are bent and hands are at chest height. Exhale and push hands away from body. Inhale as you relax to starting position.

Standing Back Rows with Tubing

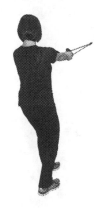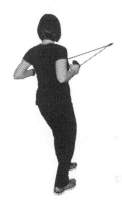

Attach tubing in middle of door hinge. Face door and step back, keeping arms straight, until tube has tension. Inhale in the relaxed position. Exhale as you pull arms back. Use the back muscles more than the arms. Keep shoulders down and relaxed. Inhale as you return to starting position.

Lunge Dive

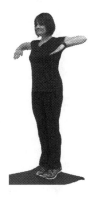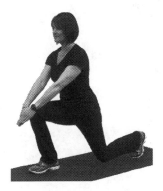

Begin by holding arms at shoulder height, pull elbows back

with palms facing down in a dive format. As you lunge forward, press arms forward as if diving into a pool. Keep head looking out and shoulders back. The body will lean slightly at a 45-degree angle. As you step in to the lunge, keep the knee over the ankle. Press back to a standing position. Alternate legs for the required number of reps.

Front Side Lateral Combination

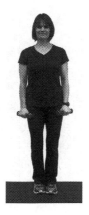 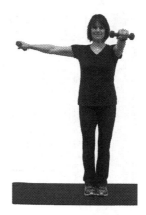

Standing or kneeling in correct postural position, abs in, feet (knees) shoulder-width apart (if standing, knees slightly bent), begin with the arms hanging at side. Lift the dumbbell to above shoulder height with right arm, keeping left arm at side. Lower right arm and repeat action with left arm. Continue to alternate for the required number of reps.

Segment 3: Core

Perform three sets of 10 reps of each exercise. Repeat circuit for 5 to 7 minutes.

Arm and Leg Balance

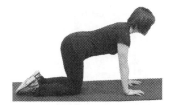 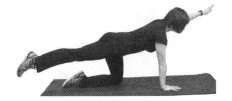

On an exercise mat, from starting position on all-fours, keep back straight. Exhale as you raise right arm until it is even with shoulder and simultaneously lift left leg until even with hip. Hold this position for two to three counts. (Focus on holding kegel throughout movement. If it drops, pause and draw it back in and continue to finish repetitions.) Repeat on other side. Alternate for the required number of reps.

Russian Twist

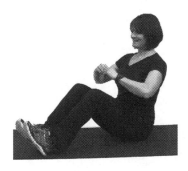 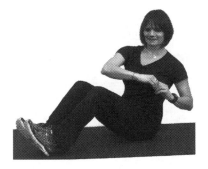

Sit straight and tall, knees bent. Lean back slightly, while maintaining correct posture. Clasp hands together at chest height. Holding ab muscles in, rotate slowly from side to side.

Low-Ab Roll

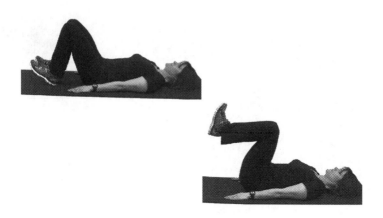

Lay face up with knees bent, feet flat on floor, arms extended to sides, pressing palms into mat to help stabilize the movement. Draw the navel into the body, contracting the abdominal muscles lift feet up off the mat drawing the knees toward the mid-line of the body. Once the knees reach the mid-line, slowly lower the feet back to the mat. Exhale as you draw the knees up. Inhale as you relax.

NOTE: Modifications – bring one knee up to center while leaving the other foot flat to the mat.

Segment 4: Cardio

From the One-Minute Movement Starters (TOOL NO. 3), select four. Perform the four exercises for a total of 10 minutes. Increase if desired. For example, you may count reps, such as set of 20 reps each exercise, or you may time the exercise, such as 30 seconds each exercise. Repeat the circuit for 10 minutes or walk, run, or bike ride.

Cool Down

Walk for three to five minutes, until heart rate returns to 120 or less. Next, relax, stretch, and perform deep breathing.

Basic Core & Advanced Level Workout Instructions

The following workouts are formulated for three levels. Level 1 is the Basic Core, which is for everyone. Before moving up a level, I highly recommend investing time in these Basic Core exercises. Maintain focus on structural stability, such as holding the navel in towards the backbone; pelvic bone pulled towards the navel; kegel and hips square (do not lean on one hip). Maintain a correct posture throughout the movements. Level 2, for the moderate fitness level, uses Level 1 and 2 programs to formulate the workout plan. Level 3, for the advanced exerciser, uses Level 1 through Level 3 programs to formulate the workout plan.

Don't be hesitant about mixing it up. The key to a sustainable workout plan is variety and not feeling stuck. For example, if bored with counting reps, perform the exercises for a period of time, such as three sets of 45 seconds or a timed ladder starting with 30 seconds of each exercise, then 45 seconds, ending with 60 seconds. Rest as needed and work your way back down the ladder.

A typical ladder would look like this: 30-45-60 seconds, rest for one to two minutes, 60-45-30 seconds. For less intensity, do only one 60-second set in the middle.

Here are other options:

- Three sets of 30 seconds each exercise, gradually building to 60 seconds of each exercise;
- Do a repetition count, 20 reps; 15 reps; 10 reps; or
- For a greater challenge, do a 50-rep challenge or a 100-rep (of each exercise on the chosen workout program) challenge (for advanced level only).

I strongly suggest that you accompany all workout plans with activities you love. Just because you did one of these workouts in the morning, doesn't mean you can't enjoy an activity in the afternoon or evening, such as walking or wading in the pool, jumping on a rebounder, dancing, yoga, flow and stretch. I'm not suggesting you work out two times a day. I am recommending an active lifestyle, one where you are not "afraid" to burn energy on what you love and enjoy. Be active for your body, because it desires movement. It was made for it. Before starting any exercise program, consult your physician.

TOOL NO. 5:

Basic Core Routine 1

Do three non-consecutive sets of 10 to 20 reps of each exercise. Rest after each set. Utilize deep breathing throughout the movements. Focus on the muscle group being worked by bringing the mind into the muscle.

Shoulder Bridge:

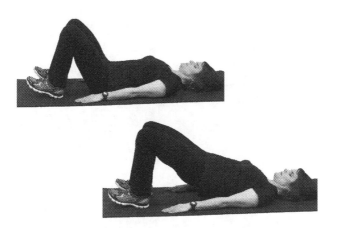

Lie on back with knees bent, feet flat on floor. Raise toes and dig heels into floor. Squeeze the glutes as you raise the hips off the floor. Hold for two seconds and return hips to floor.

Straight Leg Raise:

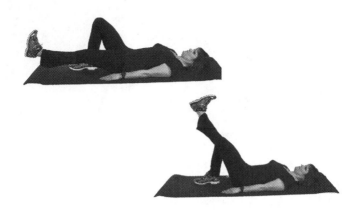

Lie on back with one knee bent and the other extended parallel to floor. Raise leg to knee height while holding abs in, then lower leg back to floor.

Eagle Abs:

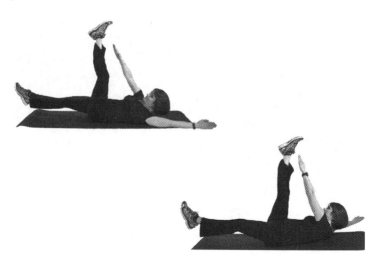

Lie with legs extended out and arms extended over head. Engage the abs. Raise right leg and touch with left arm. Return to starting position. Switch to other side. Alternate back and forth for required number of reps. Tip: Keep the heel pressed into the floor while the other leg extends straight up.

Prone Swim with Extension:

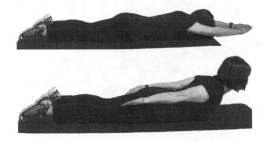

Lie on stomach, arms extended over head. Holding abs in, lift arms off floor and swing them to the lower back. At the same time, raise upper body off floor into an extended position. Relax and swing arms back to starting position.

4-Point Straight Leg Hip Extension:

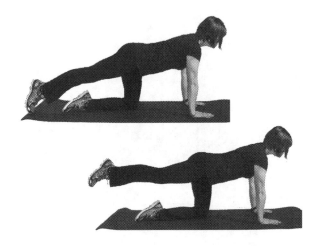

In a four-point stance, drop down onto forearms. Extend one leg back. Using glute muscle, raise leg. Lower to floor. Repeat, alternating legs.

Side-Lying Leg Raise:

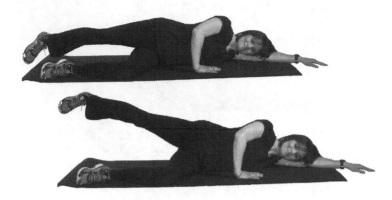

Lie on the side, bottom knee bent at 90-degree angle, and top leg extended. Raise and lower leg at slow pace. Keep hips on top of one another. Do not let top hip roll back. Reverse and repeat with other leg.

TOOL NO. 6:

Basic Core Routine 2

Perform 10 reps of each exercise. Rest one minute, repeat four to five times. Keep track of the number of sets on a workout calendar. Gradually increase to five sets of 15 reps.

Modified Chest Push-Up:

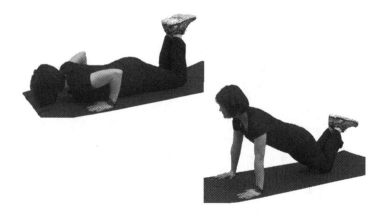

Begin in a plank position but drop the knees to the ground and pull the feet tight to the bum. Roll forward on knees to soft part above kneecaps, keeping shoulders in line above wrists. Perform push-up for specified number of times. Keep abs tight and lower body as close to floor as possible. Lead with the chest and avoid tucking in head.

Floor Jacks:

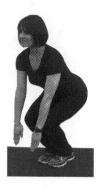 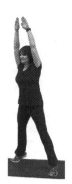

Begin with feet together in a narrow squat position. Keep the abs pulled in tight, shoulders pulled back, face forward, and arms extended to the ground. Power up, open legs to an inverted-V stance, and extend arms to the sky. Bring the legs back to a narrow stance and squat with arms reaching to ground.

Side-Plank Dip – Modified Version

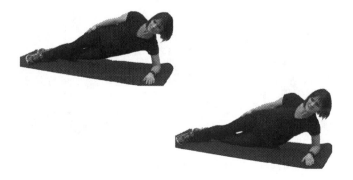

In side plank position with elbow directly under shoulder, feet staggered for balance, press body up with core maintaining the hold with only the forearm and feet to maintain position. As an alternative, bend the leg closest to the floor and press up into the plank from knee. Tap hip to floor for required number of reps. Reverse and repeat on other side.

Full Body, Bend-Over Walkout:

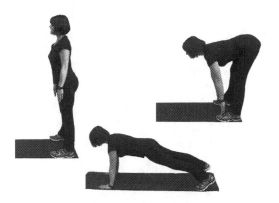

Begin in standing position with feet shoulder-width or farther apart. Engaging ab muscles, bend forward and place hands on floor. Keeping knees as straight as possible, walk hands out to form a full plank position. Maintain a tight core while holding this for two counts. Walk the hands back in towards the feet. Leading with head and shoulders, raise body to a standing position. DO NOT RAISE BODY TO A STANDING POSITION WITH A ROUNDED BACK.

Mule Kicks, Side:

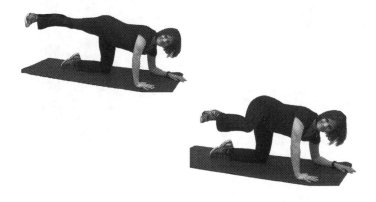

Begin in four-point stance on elbows. Draw knee up and out to side. Extend leg, toes pointed. Repeat on other side.

TOOL NO. 7:

Moderate Routine

Start with two sets of 10 reps of each exercise. Build to 15 reps then increase to three sets. Minimally rest between exercises and rest one to two minutes between sets.

Plank Pat-a-Cake:

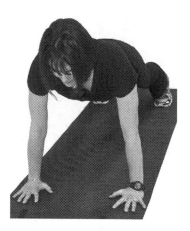 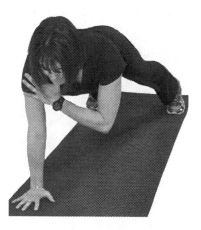

Begin in plank position, shoulders over wrists, hips at shoulder height, legs and abs tight. Begin by bringing the right hand over to slap the left shoulder then return to ground. Repeat on other side.

Ball Wall Squat:

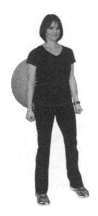
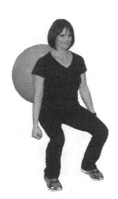

Place ball against wall at stomach height. Lean back against ball so it rests comfortably along the curve of the lower back. Place feet in front of body so that, when squatting, knees line up with ankles. Squat until hips are in line with knees. Press back to starting position by driving heels into floor and squeezing the glutes.

Ball Wall Pushups:

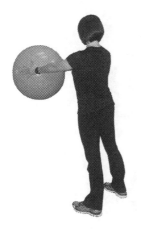
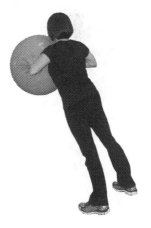

Hold ball against wall at chest height. Bend elbows until chest touches ball. Push chest away from ball back to starting position. Some alternatives: Do a one-half full body pushup or do counter pushups.

Crab Walk:

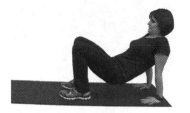 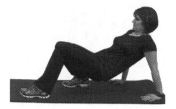

In a crab position, facing up, hands under shoulders, knees bent, lead with hands and walk the specified distance. Keep the bum off the ground as you move. Walk 10 steps forward and 10 steps back in each set.

Stationary Lunge with Bicep Curl:

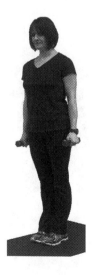 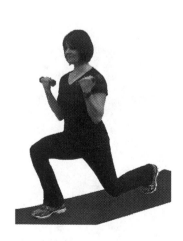

In lunge position, hold dumbbells in hands. Bend knees, curl arms up to shoulders. Using legs and glutes, push up to standing position, extending arms to sides. Repeat on other leg.

Back-Seated Back Pull with Tubing:

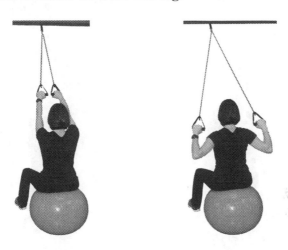

Place tubing in top of door hinge. Face the door, take hold of handles, and sit on floor or on a ball. Begin by inhaling and extending arms up. Then, exhale while pulling elbows down to ribcage. Keep arms out to sides. Inhale while returning to starting position.

Plank Mountain Climb:

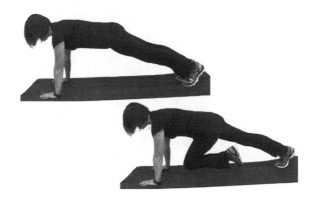

From extended plank position, shoulders over wrists, abs tight and pulled in, glutes engaged, draw knee to chest, and quickly alternate with other knee. Use quick movement as knees are drawn forward. Drawn-in foot does not touch the ground.

Standard Jumping Jacks:

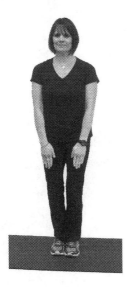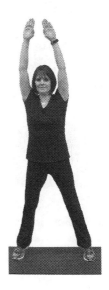

Always keep abs tight to support body. For low impact, step one foot at a time out to side.

TOOL NO. 8:

Advanced Routine 1

Perform routine as a timed ladder of 30-45-60-45-30 seconds. This means perform each exercise in the first set for 30 seconds; in the second set for 45 seconds; third set for 60 seconds; fourth set for 45 seconds; and fifth set for 60 seconds. Minimally rest between exercises and rest one minute between sets. Before starting any exercise program, consult your physician.

Legs/Hindu Squat:

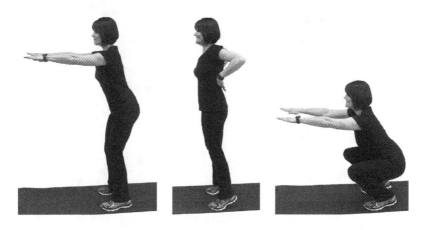

Begin standing with feet flat and arms extended in front. With abs tight and pulled in, lower body to a squat stance, leading arms with pointed fingers in a backward rotation while rising up on toes. As arms rotate to extend out, return to standing, flat-footed position.

Belly Blaster:

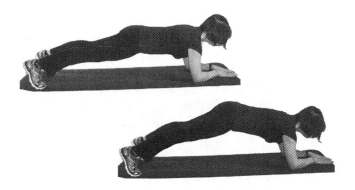

From a forearm plank position, crunch abs with a small rise to the hips and release. Maintain good form throughout exercise.

Double-Time Back Rows without Weights:

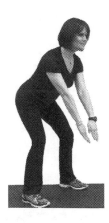
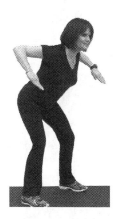

Bend forward in a back row position. Back is flat, abs in, glutes engaged to support lower back. Arms extended down in front. Pull arms back, bending elbows towards the sky. Get comfortable with movement before you perform at a double-time rate. Move through the exercise as quickly as possible, maintaining correct form.

Plank Step-Ups:

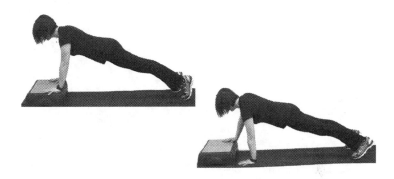

Begin in a plank position, hands on bench. Position feet shoulder-width apart. Position hips at shoulder height, hold abdominals in tight to support back. Drop down with right hand, then left, step up with right, and then left. Now switch, drop down with left hand first, then right, and then left. Continue to alternate hands for the designated time. It is important to maintain form. If unable to continue, stop exercise and rest before completing the required number of reps.

Gorilla Squats:

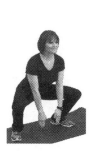
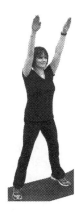

Begin in a wide stance, toes pointed out. Keeping back straight and shoulders back, lower body as low as possible. Goal is to touch floor with fingertips. Next, rise to a standing position, raising arms overhead, and reaching up onto toes. Keep abs in and squeeze glutes as you stand.

Full Body/ Straight Leg Bridge:

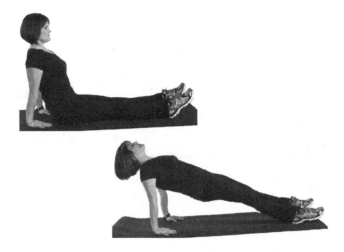

Sit with legs straight out. Place hands behind with fingertips facing forward. Dig heels into floor as you squeeze the glutes and raise the hips from the floor to chest height. Return to starting position.

TOOL NO. 9:

Advanced Routine 2

Perform using a rep ladder of 20-15-10-10-15-20 repetitions, meaning in the ladder's first rung, do 20 reps; on the second, 15 reps; on the third, 10 reps; on the fourth, 10 reps; on the fifth, 15 reps; and on the sixth, 20 reps. Modify rep count as needed to adjust to your particular fitness level.

Lunge with Suicide Tap-Downs:

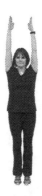 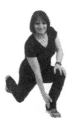

Begin in a standing position, arms overhead. Step out with right foot at a 45-degree angle. While stepping out, lunge, bending front knee over shoelaces and dropping hips. Tap down with left hand as close to ground as possible. Quickly push back to standing position, and while making a vertical jump, extend arms high overhead. Land lightly on balls of feet. Repeat on left side.

Back/Plank Rows with Dumbbells:

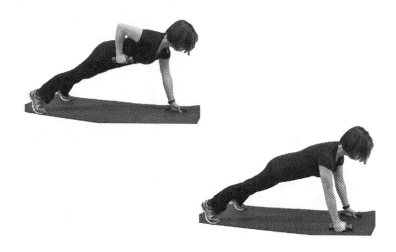

Position body in plank position, aligning shoulders with wrists and navel pulled in to backbone. Place knees toward top of thigh, contracting the quadriceps. Draw dumbbell towards ribcage as you would in a typical dumbbell back row, pause, and then return arm to starting position. Alternate arms for required time. Maintain proper form throughout movement. Stop and rest, if needed.

Snow Boarders, High Impact:

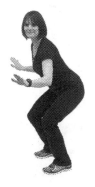
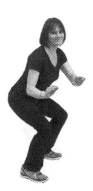

Begin in a low squat position. Raise body up using the hips and thighs, then, in midair, turn body to face other direction. Land body in a low squat position. Continue jumping and turning for required amount of time. This is an advanced exercise, so use caution if you have back and knee issues. Choose a low impact exercise from one of the moderate workouts, if this proves to be too advanced.

Wide Grip Pushups:

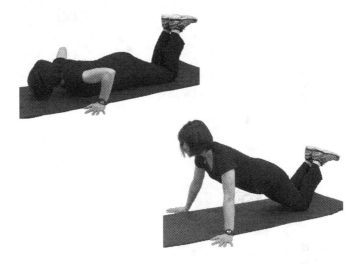

Begin in an extended plank position with hands in wide grip (hands outside the chest wall, angled out). Keeping the shoulders over the wrists, abs tight, and glutes engaged, slowly lower body to the ground for a pushup, and then extend, returning to starting position.

Power Jacks (Squats):

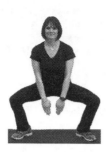 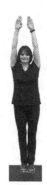

Begin in a wide squat with hips low. Power up and bring feet together as arms reach overhead. Jump up and land in a wide squat position, bringing arms down to center to complete the exercise.

Arnold Shoulder Press:

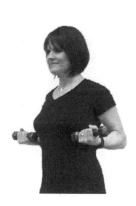 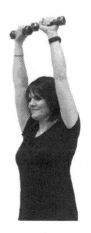

Hold dumbbell curled tight at chest height. Push dumbbell overhead while turning the dumbbell to face outward. Return to starting position by turning dumbbell back inward, and lower to chest height, keeping dumbbell curled. As you do this, draw the shoulder blades back to contract the rear deltoid.

TOOL NO. 10:

Back Health & Maintenance

"My aching back!" On any given day, more than 30 million Americans complain of lower back pain, and back pain is one of the most cited reasons for calling in too sick to work. An estimated $50 billion a year is spent on doctor visits, medications, surgeries, and therapies that address pains in the back. Some back pain is the result of a serious medical condition such as kidney or other infections, fractures, cancer, or arthritis, but the source of most complaints are not as easily explained. Poor posture, obesity, inactivity, uncomfortable shoes, and sleeping on a worn-out mattress can contribute to chronic back pain. So can anxiety.

For a number of years, back pain was my constant companion. The more I thought about it, the more I feared it, and the more I feared the pain, the more intense it became. The pain became a debilitating self-prophecy.

"What will I do if this gets worse?"

"What if this never goes away?"

"Can I get through another day?"

Realizing these toxic thoughts intensified the fear of pain, and, in so doing, made it unbearable, I refused to connect emotional feelings with pain. To this end, I adopted a course of action and a favorite saying. Acknowledging pain, I took a deep breath, lived with the pain in that moment, relaxed, and moved on, saying, "Hmm, that was interesting." Of course, the pain was there, at times it was intense, but I accepted it, because I believed it could not be worse in the next moment. "Hmm, that was interesting" was preferable to "Oh, that hurt."

Correct posture and alignment, plus a back maintenance routine that increases muscle strength and overall flexibility and mobility, can go a long way to diminish pain. Here is a posture tip: Stand with feet several inches apart. Slightly bending the knees, shift your body weight to the forefeet, the heels lightly placed on the floor. Elongate the spine by allowing the tail bone to "drop" towards the floor and the crown of the head to "reach" for the sky. Draw back the shoulders and slightly "drop" the shoulder blades into your back pockets. Pull in the navel to complete the posture exercise.

I've provided five "back maintenance" exercises that may not necessarily cure back pain, but may offer some relief. Use these routines to strengthen back muscles and practice good posture. Before starting any exercise program, consult your physician.

Cobra Stretch:

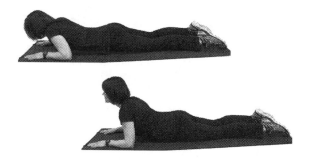

Starting in a face-down, prone position with forearms under the chest, engage the glutes, pull in the abs, and gradually raise the upper torso. Hold for 10 to 15 seconds. Repeat 10 times a day. As a variation, build up the flexibility to fully extend arms during the stretch.

Shoulder Bridge:

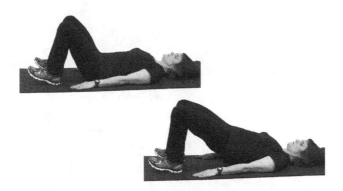

On back with knees bent and feet flat on floor, raise toes while digging heels into floor. Next, squeeze the glutes while raising hips off the floor. Hold for 5 to 10 seconds and return hips to floor. Repeat 15 to 20 times.

Arm & Leg Balance:

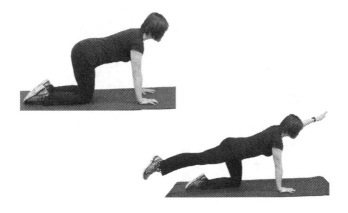

Starting in a four-point stance, contract the abdominal muscles by pulling the pelvis to the navel. Inhale and extend the right arm and left leg. Exhale. Hold position for 5 seconds. Return to four-stance starting position. Repeat by extending left arm and right leg. Repeat 10 to 15 times.

Modified Side Plank:

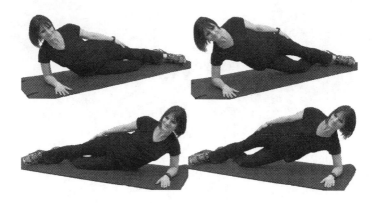

Side Plank Dip - Modified version

Level 1 bottom leg is bent underneath you so that when you press up you are on the side of the leg.

Begin in a side lying position, propped up on forearm with the hips lined up one on top of the other. Pull the abs in strong and engage the glutes (bum), press the body up off the ground so that you are balancing on the forearm and feet. Keep body long and straight. Hold for 5 counts; Repeat 15-20 x on each side.

Advanced version

Foot placement:

Level 2: both legs extended with the feet staggered.

Level 3: most difficult – feet are stacked one on top of the other.

TOOL NO. 11:

The Truth About Supplements

If the foods we eat make us who we are, the nutritional supplements we select strengthen our immunity in the battle against premature aging. For many people, especially individuals who may skip meals or otherwise are not eating enough whole foods, or anyone who wants the best for their bodies, nutritional supplements are essential for a longer, healthier life. On the cellular level, cells tend to malfunction when they are either deficient in proper nutrition or are exposed to toxic chemicals, namely the pesticides, fungicides, and herbicides used by mega-farms to increase yields and profits.

Eating organically grown, whole foods is the best way to avoid harmful pesticides, fungicides, and herbicides, but despite our best efforts to eat healthy foods, we need to supplement our diets with essential vitamins and minerals. Before purchasing a multi-vitamin at the grocery, be aware that all supplements are not the same. Most, particularly those sold in grocery stores, are manufactured in chemical factories from fossil fuels such as coal tar, petroleum products, and rocks. Cheap to make and profitable to sell, these kinds of supplements are difficult to digest or are not digestible at all.

Supplements made from natural, plant-sourced vitamins, minerals, and glyconutrients are best, and that is why I recommend the health, wellness, weight, and fitness products manufactured by

Mannatech. For more than two decades, this U.S.-based company's "Real Food Technology" solutions, backed by $20 million in research, more than seventy worldwide patents, and certified by NSF International, has made a difference for millions. Mannatech was a pioneer in identifying ground-breaking glyconutrients, dietary supplement ingredients containing beneficial amounts of polysaccharides, compounds recognized to strengthen the immune system, improve digestion, and enhance cognitive and memory function.

In recent years, research scientists have determined that optimal cellular function depends on the presence of glycoproteins, cell surface sugar structures essential for a healthy immune system. When the body has a lack of certain glycoproteins, its immune system cells are unable to discern healthy cells from those that need to be nourished, repaired, regulated, or destroyed. Mannatech's powerful Ambrotose supplements provide one of the most potent and healthy mixes of glyconutrients available to support immune function. For example, the Ambrotose selection of supplements contain plant extracts, antioxidant compounds such as vitamins C and E, a very pure aloe vera gel powder, and the sea vegetable Undaria pinnatifida, a rich source of omega-3 fatty acid, calcium, iodine, thiamine, and niacin. This combination of natural ingredients supports the immune system, boosts energy, and nourishes cellular function.

Other Mannatech nutritional supplements specifically address heart health, overall levels of energy, digestion, the secretion of critical hormones, and the maintenance of blood sugar levels, especially following intense workouts. Mannatech products are available from the company's independent associates or directly from the company at mannatch.com.

Ashly Torian is an Independent Associate of Mannatech Incorporated and is the daughter of J. Stanley Fredrick, Chairman of the Board of Mannatech Incorporated.

TOOL NO. 12:

Successful Grocery Shopping

Fat-charged packaged foods, frozen pizzas, ready-to-eat frozen dinners, deli meats, sandwich cookies and more comprise the standard American diet, abbreviated as SAD. That acronym is not a coincidence. Neither is the design of most supermarkets that groups foods and snacks in long aisles, notably cookies in one, breakfast cereals in another, and a gargantuan pile of sodas near the center of the store. In this convenience-friendly environment, grocery shopping is a definite challenge, particularly if you intend to avoid the SAD way of eating.

Break the SAD cycle by purchasing and preparing healthy food choices. Warning, patience and mental adjustments are required, but with practice, old habits can be replaced with the fine art of healthy shopping. Start with a plan and a list. Never again push a cart through a grocery without a meal plan and a list of your required ingredients. Determine the meals you will prepare in the upcoming week and make a grocery list accordingly. Eat before shopping. A hungry stomach almost always wins over a disciplined mind.

Inside the store, push your cart around the market's perimeter. In most grocery layouts, the perimeter displays the perishables such as fresh fruits and vegetables, meats, and dairy offerings.

After shopping the perimeter, head to frozen foods for out-of-season fruits and vegetables. Finally, hit the aisles for seasonings, oils, nuts, seeds, olives, and organic canned or dried beans. If a packaged food is part of your upcoming recipes, look for those containing three or fewer ingredients and no or minimal preservatives.

Avoid "detours" by ignoring the alluring packaging of ready-to-eat dinners and boxed products. The beautiful photography seldom resembles the meal inside and always fails to picture the unhealthy, fatty, high-sodium contents. Like double-stuffed cookies, these foods are lovely temptations. Stay away.

On your grocery days, replace SAD with HAPPY:

- **H**andpick healthy foods.
- **A**void detours and temptations.
- **P**lan your meals.
- **P**repare a grocery list.
- **Y**ield to traffic headed to the cookies and go straight to the checkout line.

TOOL NO. 13:

Quick & Easy Dinner Recipes

Easy-to-prepare, nutritious foods using wholesome, fresh ingredients, hands down beat prepackaged processed and frozen foods. There is no need to sacrifice quality for convenience. Select from these quick recipes and search for others online. In the **END Zone**, you can prepare tasty and healthy meals in a snap.

Chicken Quesadillas
- Sprouted tortillas
- Chicken breast—prepared ahead & sliced
- Goat cheese or feta cheese
- Jalapenos and onions (optional)
- Avocado slices
- Coconut oil or REAL butter for toasting

Spread a small amount of coconut oil or butter on one side of each tortilla. Place one tortilla in hot skillet (butter side down). Add chicken and cheese on open face. Lay other tortilla on top with butter side up. Cook until toasted and heated through. Flip. Toast other side. Serve with fresh salsa and avocado slices.

Turkey Burgers
- Turkey patty – prepared ahead

- Sprouted bread OR Iceberg lettuce
- Sautéed mushrooms

Heat turkey patty, toast sprouted bread, sauté mushrooms in coconut oil or olive oil. Assemble and enjoy! Serve with veggie cup (cauliflower, celery, and red cabbage mixed with olive oil, sea salt, and a squeeze of lemon).

Bean Salad
- 2 to 3 types of beans (kidney, garbanzo, green, yellow wax, black-eyed peas)
- Chopped grape tomatoes
- Chopped zucchini
- Chopped green olives
- Green, yellow and red peppers (optional)
- Shaved parmesan cheese (optional)
- Other ingredients as desired
- Serve cold or at room temperature. Make once and enjoy several times during the week. Can be added to a green salad.

Chicken Spaghetti
- Spaghetti squash
- Organic chunky tomato and herb sauce
- Chicken breast prepared ahead
- Portabella mushrooms

Bake spaghetti squash at 350° for 45 minutes. Slice in half, partially cool, remove seeds. Squash is ready when strings easily pull away from rind. If not ready, place open side up in a baking dish, brush inside with olive oil or a little butter, and continue baking. When cooked, scrape out noodles. Store up to a week in refrigerator. Cook chicken in water. Sauté mushrooms in olive oil or coconut oil until nearly tender, then add chicken for flavor. Add seasonings, if desired. Stir in tomato sauce and heat until hot. Pour tomato sauce and chicken mixture over spaghetti squash for the most delightful spaghetti ever! Enjoy!

Ashly's Skillet Dinner Mix! (My favorite!)
* Sautéed mushrooms
* Frozen butternut squash
* Okra
* Fresh rosemary
* Chicken cooked ahead in coconut oil or olive oil
* Parmesan cheese (grated)

Place vegetables on a cookie sheet. Season with rosemary to taste. Bake at 350° until tender. Add chicken and top with grated parmesan. YUMMY!

Lettuce Rolls
* Leaf lettuce (dark green leaves) or collard greens
* Chicken or another fresh meat (no nitrates or preservatives), prepared ahead
* Cheese (sliced)
* Tomato (sliced)

Roll cooked chicken or other meat, cheese, and tomato in lettuce leaf.

Variations include:

Lettuce taco wrap with cooked fish and cabbage.

Lettuce wrap with chicken salad. (Made with fresh, cooked shredded chicken, sliced celery, onions, collard green stalk, cranberries (crushed), hummus, or honey mustard.)

Lettuce wrap with refried beans, grated cheese, picante sauce, and a little sour cream.

(To make your own refried beans, rinse pinto beans and cook to boiling with 1/4 to 1/2 teaspoon coconut oil, water to desired consistency, and salt. Cook beans until soft, then mash to a creamy consistency.)

Black Bean/Avocado Salad
- 1 can black beans
- 1 can kidney beans
- 2 avocadoes
- 15 green olives (queen), sliced
- 15 kalamata olives, sliced
- ½ jicima, chopped

Combine in a bowl, toss with Himalayan sea salt, and enjoy! Yields 4 servings.

Squash Salad
- 4 zucchini squash, spiral sliced
- ½ jicima, julienne sliced
- 1 butternut squash, spiral sliced or julienne sliced
- 2 Roma tomatoes
- Parmesan cheese
- Himalayan sea salt to taste

After slicing, combine in a bowl and toss veggies with parmesan cheese and Himalayan sea salt.

More mealtime ideas:

Traditional Dinner Night
Bake chicken, fish, or turkey. Serve with quinoa (seasoned with sautéed onions, portabella mushrooms, and Himalayan sea salt) plus grilled asparagus, or other favorite veggie.

Taco Night
Combine chopped tomato, avocado, black olives, onions, peppers, and either black beans or pinto beans to make black bean salsa. Set aside. Cover sprouted corn tortilla with shaved parmesan cheese and warm in oven. Remove from oven, and top with black bean salsa.

Salad with Everything

Chop your favorite veggies. I love to add shaved butternut squash (uncooked) to enhance any salad with scrumptious flavor. Add spring mixed greens and arugula. Top with parmesan cheese and Himalayan sea salt mixed with olive oil. For protein, add cooked chicken tenders or beans.

Omelets

A family favorite, breakfast for dinner, made with omelets filled with anything you like. Use goat, sheep, or feta cheese. Get creative.

Spaghetti Squash Delight

Spaghetti squash, garbanzo beans, Italian parsley, olive oil, and Himalayan sea salt.

Caramelize garbanzo beans in sea salt and olive oil. Next, add cooked spaghetti squash and heat through. Stir in chopped Italian parsley. Enjoy!

Skillet Dinner in a Flash

Combine spaghetti squash, butternut squash, or sweet potatoes to make a skillet dinner in a flash. Simply add one or two other veggies, cooked meat or beans, and seasonings for a delightful meal.

Preparing meals is easier when you plan a menu. Purchase meats on Saturday and cook on Sunday to be ready for the coming week. You will reduce prep time and have meals on the table in a flash.

Conclusion

The journey to sustainable fitness and health is as much about counting on your ability to discern what you decide is a purposeful life as it is about counting calories and exercise repetitions. Rather than quantify success based on pounds and inches lost, measure happiness based on living the life you were meant to live. To designate your ideal level of fitness, decide what you need your body to do, because, in the **END Zone**, you can reshape attitudes and beliefs in the image of the person you want to become. You can adopt a transformative lifestyle, one that places you in charge of your future.

Embrace the body you have. That's your starting point. From this moment forward, love the body you have to get the body you want.

Nourish it with wholesome foods and beneficial movement.

Digest the world around you in harmony and balance. Replace toxic thoughts with affirmative ones. Substitute fears and anxieties with truth and fact.

Mindfully live each day, and I will join you in the **END Zone**.

Ashly Torian

As founder and owner of Bio-Balance, Ashly began her Holistic Eating and Body Image coaching business in 1991, committed to inspiring others to live a fulfilling, joy-filled life. Bio-Balance was born out of Ashly's passion for fitness and healthy living seeded with her own personal challenges with anxiety, weight and body image issues.

Ashly works with those who desire to set themselves FREE from the pain and struggle they experience with food and body. For some it is a roller coaster ride of diet and emotions, for others it is seeking false perfection. Ashly holds a safe place for you to freely express and release what is holding you hostage.

Ashly is a Texan, receiving her Bachelor of Science degree in Adult Corporate Fitness from Abilene Christian University, followed by training at the Institute for the Psychology of Eating, the world's leading school in Nutritional Psychology where she received her certification as an Eating Psychology Coach. In addition, Ashly is a nationally recognized ACE certified personal fitness trainer and behavior change coach; as well as a recognized IDEA Elite personal fitness trainer with thousands of individual and corporate exercise programs to her credit.

Ashly guides her clients to focus on their highest goal, not the small goal of how much weight they can lose this week, but their highest goal; their reason for being. When this is the focal point, they can then embrace a healthy lifestyle that empowers them to make nourishing choices about food, body and life.

Visit www.ashlytorian.com to discover resources, view the cheering section about Ashly, and see how investing in YOU can change your life.

About Jim Waldsmith

Jim Waldsmith is a professional writer who works with Fortune 500 companies and executives. A former news reporter, editor, and news director, this award-winning journalist is an accomplished speech writer and producer. His company, Jim Waldsmith's Creative Arts, LLC, is located in Columbus, Ohio. Previous books include *Make it a Winning Day* and *A Regular Guy's Guide to Success* about Wendy's R. David Thomas and Dave Longaberger, founder of The Longaberger Company. Jim can be reached at www.jwca.com.

Printed in the United States
By Bookmasters